Some Spoons Are Worth Spending

Practical Energy Conservation Strategies to Live Your Best Life With Myasthenia Gravis

Dr. Liz Plowman

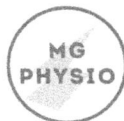

MG
PHYSIO

Some Spoons Are Worth Spending: Practical Energy Conservation Strategies to Live Your Best Life with Myasthenia Gravis

Copyright © 2024 by Liz Plowman

Published by Liz Plowman

Edited and formatted by Joanne Martin

Front and back cover art and design by GetCovers

ISBN (paperback): 979-8-9907745-0-6

ISBN (e-book): 979-8-9907745-2-0

This book is a work of nonfiction. While every effort has been made to ensure the accuracy and completeness of the information contained herein, the author and publisher assume no responsibility for errors, inaccuracies, omissions, or any inconsistencies herein.

❄

Disclaimer: This book is NOT, nor shall it be construed in any way as, medical advice. The information, guides, and tips contained in these pages are designed to be general suggestions only. Please take your personal circumstances, health status, and needs into consideration before incorporating any of the suggestions in this book. Consult with your healthcare team with any questions you may have before making any changes.

To the memory of my mother, Marilyn—
tremendous nurse,
tireless entrepreneur,
mighty ALS warrior,
my biggest fan,
and the magic behind the most delicious chocolate cake on the planet.

I love you, Mom.

I miss you.

❄

Contents

Author's Note   vii

1. Why Spoons Matter   1
2. Energy Budget   4
3. Assistive Devices   28
4. Life Hacks   44
5. Exercising Safely   60
6. Working   83
7. Traveling   104
8. Asking for Help   120
9. In Case of Emergency   132
10. Grace, Compassion, and Self Care   145

Acknowledgments   151
Additional Resources   153
About the Author   155

Author's Note

First things first... *Thank you!*

Thank you for picking up this book. Thank you for refusing to accept the status quo in life with Myasthenia Gravis (MG). Thank you for being brave enough to do something about finding a better quality of life for yourself.

Well done!

❄

Who I Am

While we will get to know each other better as you read through these pages, I'd like to ease your concerns about who I am and why I am qualified to write this book.

My name is Liz. Nice to meet you! I am a physical therapist (or physiotherapist, if you are outside the United States). I work exclusively with people with MG, and I have MG myself. So, I live what you live every single day. My personal and professional goal is to take my clinical expertise combined with my personal experience and make life with MG just a little bit easier and a whole lot more enjoyable.

What This Book IS

This book is exactly what the cover says it is: a collection of practical energy conservation strategies to help you live your BEST LIFE with MG.

Over the years of working with clients with MG (not to mention living through it myself), I have compiled a collection of strategies, tips, tricks, and hacks. My clients have frequently encouraged me to put my educational material together in a book, so I've done just that.

This book is designed to be a helpful guide to make living with MG more manageable and to help you have energy left over to spend on things that truly matter to you and bring you joy.

What This Book IS NOT

It's easier if I make a list for this one...

- **This book is NOT, nor shall it be construed in any way as, medical advice.** (My lawyer made me write that.)
- **This book is NOT a cure for MG**. Believe me, if I had my hands on the cure for MG, I'd be first in line. And this book would be a lot more expensive.
- **This book is NOT an individualized treatment for MG**. There is absolutely no way I can do that in a book. The information, guides, and tips contained in these pages are designed to be general suggestions only. Please take your personal circumstances, health status, and needs into consideration before incorporating any of the

suggestions in this book. **Also—and I cannot emphasize this enough—consult with your healthcare team about any questions before making any changes.**

How to Use This Book

How you use this book is truly up to you. I've designed it to be read from start to finish, but each chapter can stand alone. So, if you are a cover-to-cover reader, go for it. If you are a picker-and-chooser, then skip around and read the sections that appeal most to you. If there are sections that don't apply to you, feel free to skip them.

The book is front-loaded. That is to say, the bulk of the information is provided in the first few chapters, and more detailed and situation-specific information is provided in later chapters. I recommend reading chapters 1 through 4 first and then skipping to chapters or sections that apply to you personally. (But please don't skip the final chapter.)

What are you waiting for? Grab a spoon and dig in!

Chapter 1

Why Spoons Matter

WHEN I WAS ABOUT SIX MONTHS INTO MY LIFE WITH Myasthenia Gravis (MG) and dealing with the mobility loss, change in my functional ability, and identity changes that came with it, I bit the bullet and decided to ask my physician for an accessible parking placard to make outings a tiny bit less exhausting. I had finally started using a cane at that point and enjoyed the increased freedom and ease of mobility that it gave me. I was ready for more freedom.

My family physician, who had looked after me since I was two years old, sat across from me at my dad's kitchen table. (He also happened to be my dad's neighbor, and they swapped swimming pool maintenance tips. Ah, the joys of a small town.) My then 14-month-old daughter was at my feet, playing with various plastic containers she had purloined from a kitchen cabinet.

"I won't use it all the time," I began. "I'll only park in a handicapped spot if I'm really symptomatic."

He frowned. "Liz, let me ask you something. Would you rather spend your energy playing with your daughter or walking across a parking lot?"

I smiled. "Point taken."

And that point has stayed with me in the years since. With MG, energy conservation is an essential part of management. Phrases like "save your spoons" are repeated frequently in the MG community, but I ask, to what end? While yes, in order to stay healthy, people living with MG need to avoid overexerting, but there's a purpose in conserving energy beyond energy conservation for energy conservation's sake. We save "spoons" for the activities that *really matter*.

That conversation with my family doctor was a turning point for me. Though asking for help often goes against my nature, I realized that being strategic with my energy would allow me to participate more fully in the activities that bring me joy. As I drove away from the DMV that same day with a bright blue plastic parking placard in hand, I thought more about his question. I realized that in the months since my MG diagnosis, I had been so focused on trying to maintain my previous active lifestyle that I was missing out on precious moments with my daughter.

In my "former life" (read: before MG), I was constantly on the go —working long hours as a military physical therapist, going to the gym, and hosting dinner parties and game nights. Now, even a short trip to the grocery store could wipe me out for hours. I was still clinging to my identity as the energetic, high-achieving woman I used to be, not yet ready to accept the new limitations MG had placed on me.

But my doctor was right. Chasing the ghost of my former self was neither possible nor wise anymore. If I insisted on expending all my limited energy on basic tasks I could now only accomplish with assistance, I wouldn't have anything left over for my family, my profession, or me.

Each time I caught myself starting to do something the harder way out of habit or stubbornness, I would hear his voice in my head: "Would you rather spend your energy on this or on your daughter?" The answer was obvious.

That makeshift appointment at my dad's kitchen table marked a shift in my mindset. I started to look at my life through the lens of energy conservation and prioritization. Instead of clinging to who I used to be, I asked myself who I wanted to become in this new reality. I realized that while some things would inevitably change, the core of who I was remained. I was still a physical therapist passionate about helping others, a wife who loved cooking elaborate meals with her husband, and a mom who delighted in every giggle and milestone. With strategic planning and the support of my loved ones, I could find new ways to engage in activities meaningful to me.

My husband and I devised a system where he took over more physically demanding household tasks, and I focused my energy on caring for our daughter. (A son joined us two years later.) We switched to more convenient, simple meals during the week, saving our epic culinary creations for restful weekends. And, probably the hardest of all, I asked for (and accepted) help from friends and family. My husband's parents were happy to drive me to appointments when my double vision was raging and babysit so that I could rest.

So, while the primary focus of this book is strategies for energy conservation and working smarter, not harder, with MG, please keep in mind that my ultimate goal is to teach you to conserve energy on the activities that don't matter as much so that you have the energy to spend on the activities that are truly important. As you read through these chapters, think about what or *whom* you save your spoons for.

Some spoons are worth spending.

Chapter 2

Energy Budget

THE JOURNEY WITH MYASTHENIA GRAVIS (MG) IS INDEED a challenging one. You may have days when you feel like you're trudging through a thick, muddy swamp, every step heavy and laborious. The fatigue might sometimes seem insurmountable, like a mountain peak shrouded in clouds. But remember, every mountain has a summit that can be reached, and even the muddiest swamp clears to reveal solid ground.

Understanding your energy levels is one of the most essential "life hacks" when dealing with MG. Just like a car, your body operates on "fuel," and with MG, it's as if your fuel tank doesn't always fill to the brim. Therefore, careful management of this "fuel" becomes critical. In this first chapter, we will explore the concept of energy budgeting as a practical approach to conserving energy, avoiding overexertion, and optimizing the quality of life for individuals living with MG.

❄

ENERGY BUDGETING 101

Effective management of energy levels is essential for individuals living with MG to maintain functional independence and quality of life. Fatigue and weakness can significantly impact daily activities, making it crucial to prioritize energy conservation and optimize energy expenditure. By incorporating energy budgeting techniques into daily routines, individuals with MG can minimize symptoms, enhance well-being, and improve overall quality of life.

Several analogies can help illustrate the concept of energy budgeting. The Spoon Theory, popularized within the chronic illness community, likens energy to a finite number of spoons that must be carefully distributed throughout the day. Similarly, viewing energy expenditure through the lens of financial budgeting or battery life can also provide helpful frameworks for understanding and implementing energy conservation strategies.

The following sections will delve deeper into energy budgeting strategies, practical tips for conserving energy, and tools for monitoring and managing energy levels effectively. By embracing the concept of energy budgeting, individuals with MG can empower themselves to navigate daily challenges with resilience, vitality, and confidence.

Spoon Theory

The Spoon Theory,[1] coined by Christine Miserandino, offers a tangible way to conceptualize the limited energy reserves of individuals with chronic illnesses, including MG. In this analogy, each day begins with a finite number of "spoons," representing units

---

1. Miserandino, C. (2013). The Spoon Theory. But You Don't Look Sick? Support for those with invisible illness or chronic illness. https://butyoudontlooksick.com/articles/written-by-christine/the-spoon-theory/

of energy available for activities. Every task, whether it's getting out of bed, showering, or preparing a meal, requires spending spoons. Once all the spoons are used up, energy depletion occurs, leading to fatigue and potential symptom worsening.

For example, imagine starting the day with twelve spoons. Getting dressed might use two spoons, preparing breakfast another two, and commuting to work another three. Only five spoons remain by midday, limiting the capacity for additional activities. The Spoon Theory encourages individuals with MG to prioritize tasks, pace themselves throughout the day, and conserve spoons for essential activities.

Financial Budgeting

Comparing energy management to financial budgeting helps individuals understand the importance of allocating resources wisely to meet daily demands without overspending. Just as one manages their finances by budgeting for expenses, individuals with MG must budget their energy for various activities.

For instance, consider someone with MG who needs to attend a social event in the evening after a long day at work. They may need to budget their energy by conserving it during the day, minimizing strenuous activities, and taking regular breaks to recharge. This approach ensures they have enough energy to enjoy the event without experiencing excessive fatigue or symptom flare-ups.

Battery Life

Viewing energy expenditure through the lens of battery life visually represents energy reserves and the need for recharging. Like electronic devices, which have a limited battery capacity that is depleted with use, individuals with MG have a finite amount of energy that diminishes throughout the day.

For instance, imagine a smartphone with a full battery in the morning. As the day progresses and the phone is used for various tasks such as calls, messages, and internet browsing, the battery level decreases. To prevent the phone from running out of power prematurely, it must be recharged periodically. Similarly, individuals with MG must prioritize activities, conserve energy, and take breaks to recharge throughout the day to avoid energy depletion and fatigue.

By utilizing these analogies, individuals with MG can better understand energy management and develop effective strategies for conserving energy, pacing themselves, and optimizing their quality of life. Whether conceptualizing energy as spoons, dollars, or battery power, the overarching goal remains the same: to live a fulfilling and balanced life while effectively managing the limitations imposed by MG.

❆

ASSESSING YOUR ENERGY LEVELS

Recognizing Fatigable Weakness as a Hallmark Sign of MG

Fatigable weakness is a characteristic feature of MG, setting it apart from other neuromuscular disorders. This symptom is marked by muscle weakness that worsens with activity and improves with rest. It's crucial to discern this pattern: initially adequate strength that diminishes with repetitive or sustained muscle use.

For example, individuals with MG might notice their ability to hold conversations dwindling during social gatherings or feel a heaviness in their arms after carrying a bag for a short distance. Everyday tasks like holding a book or lifting groceries may gradually become more challenging as muscles fatigue. These subtle changes underscore the impact of MG on daily life, prompting us to manage our energy levels proactively.

Understanding the Impact of MG on Energy Levels

MG exerts a significant toll on energy reserves due to the energy-intensive nature of compensating for muscle weakness. Even seemingly simple activities such as brushing one's teeth or climbing a flight of stairs can rapidly deplete energy stores, leaving one feeling fatigued and drained. Understanding these unique challenges involves recognizing the intricate interplay between muscle weakness, neuromuscular transmission, and metabolic demands.

In generalized MG, the hallmark fatigable muscle weakness arises from antibodies attacking acetylcholine receptors at the neuromuscular junction. This disruption impairs the ability of nerve impulses to stimulate muscle contraction, leading to inefficient muscle recruitment and increased effort required for movement.[2] Consequently, individuals with MG may experience more significant energy expenditure to compensate for weakened muscles. By grasping the underlying mechanisms, we can tailor energy management strategies to alleviate symptoms and enhance daily functioning.

Determining Your "Usable Hours"

Living with MG often means balancing activity and rest to manage symptoms effectively. Many individuals with MG tend to push themselves beyond their limits, often doing too much in a day and

---

2. U.S. Department of Health and Human Services. (2024). Myasthenia Gravis. National Institute of Neurological Disorders and Stroke. http://www.ninds.nih.gov/health-information/disorders/myasthenia-gravis

then experiencing the consequences. (Sound familiar?) Understanding your usable hours can be crucial to managing your energy and maintaining your health.

Usable hours are the amount of time each day during which a person living with a chronic condition, such as MG, can engage in activities without exacerbating their symptoms. This period varies for each individual and is determined by tracking daily activities and symptoms to identify a sustainable activity level. Usable hours exclude sleep and rest periods and are a vital measure for planning and conserving energy to manage MG effectively.

Exercise to Determine Usable Hours:

1. **Track Your Activities**: Keep a detailed record of all your activities over the course of a week. Include everything from getting up to showering, dressing, cooking, eating, taking care of children, working, driving, shopping, etc. Exclude only sleep and rest periods.
2. **Tally Your Hours**: At the end of each day, add up the total number of hours spent on these activities.
3. **Monitor Your Symptoms**: Pay close attention to how you feel both on the day of the activities and the following day. Note any patterns in symptom severity related to your activity levels.
4. **Identify Overload Days**: Identify the days when you overdid it. How many hours did you use on these days? Compare this to the days when you felt relatively good.
5. **Determine Your Good Days**: Look at the number of hours you typically use on your good days. This average can help you understand how many usable hours you have each day without overextending yourself.

For example, I find that I have around eight usable hours each day. This number can go up or down depending on how I'm feeling, the intensity of the day's activities, and my sleep quality, but on average, I have around eight. After calculating your "ballpark" daily usable hours, use this number to plan your activities and manage your energy more effectively.

Practical Tips:

- **Prioritize Tasks**: Focus on the most important tasks during your usable hours.
- **Rest Periods**: Incorporate regular rest periods into your day to avoid pushing beyond your limits.
- **Adjust as Needed**: Your usable hours might fluctuate based on your health, stress levels, and other factors. Be flexible and adjust your activities accordingly.

Understanding and respecting your usable hours is a crucial strategy for conserving energy and managing MG. Planning your days around your energy limits can improve your quality of life and reduce the risk of exacerbating your symptoms.

So, how many usable hours do you have each day?

Determining Your "Peak Hours"

Identifying your "peak hours" involves pinpointing periods of the day when your energy levels are highest and best suited to engaging in more strenuous or energy-demanding activities. Given the fluctuating nature of fatigue and weakness in MG, understanding these patterns allows you to schedule tasks during peak energy times and reserve rest for periods of low energy.

For instance, some may find their energy peaks in the morning after a restful night's sleep, making it an optimal time for tasks requiring concentration or physical exertion. Conversely, energy levels may wane in the late afternoon or evening, signaling the need for rest or relaxation. Others may find that they have a more difficult time getting going in the morning but hit a stride later in the day, making the afternoon their optimal time for scheduling more strenuous activities. Personally, I am one of the former, so I do my best to schedule my most energy-demanding tasks between 9:00 AM and 11:00 AM. I also know that any activities after 3:00 PM should be low-key, if possible. Aligning activities with these "peak hours" enables you to maximize productivity, minimize fatigue, and maintain a balanced lifestyle amidst the challenges of MG.

❄

IMPLEMENTING ENERGY CONSERVATION STRATEGIES

Identifying Energy-Intensive Activities

Identifying energy-intensive activities is the first step towards effective energy conservation for individuals with MG. You can proactively manage your energy expenditure and minimize fatigue by recognizing tasks requiring significant physical or mental effort. Some common energy-intensive activities include:

- **Physical Tasks**: Activities that involve repetitive movements, heavy lifting, or prolonged standing, such as cleaning, gardening, or carrying groceries.
- **Cognitive Tasks**: Mental activities that require concentration, problem-solving, or multitasking, such as

studying, working on complex projects, or attending meetings.

- **Emotional Tasks**: Social interactions or emotional engagements that can be draining, such as attending large gatherings, participating in heated discussions, or providing emotional support to others.

Tips for Making Activities Less Energy-Expensive

Once you have identified your energy-intensive activities, there are various strategies you can implement to make these tasks less energy-expensive and more manageable. Some practical tips include:

- **Break Tasks into Smaller Steps:** Instead of tackling a task all at once, break it down into smaller, more manageable steps. This allows for rest breaks in between and reduces the overall energy expenditure.
- **Use Assistive Devices**: Utilize assistive devices or adaptive equipment to minimize the physical effort required for tasks. For example, use a rolling cart to transport heavy items or invest in ergonomic tools to reduce muscle strain.
- **Delegate Tasks**: Whenever possible, delegate tasks to family members, friends, or hired help. Sharing responsibilities lightens the workload and conserves energy for essential activities.
- **Prioritize Tasks**: Identify the most important or time-sensitive tasks and prioritize them accordingly. Focus on completing high-priority tasks during periods of peak energy and postpone less critical activities for times when energy levels are lower.
- **Practice Mindful Movement**: Pay attention to body mechanics and movement patterns to avoid unnecessary

strain or overexertion. Use proper lifting techniques, take frequent breaks, and listen to your body's signals to prevent fatigue and injury.

- **Optimize Your Environment**: Create an environment that supports energy conservation by minimizing distractions, reducing clutter, and organizing tasks in a way that promotes efficiency. Eliminate unnecessary physical or mental barriers that may drain energy unnecessarily.

Prioritizing and Allocating Energy Resources

Prioritizing and allocating energy resources involves making conscious decisions about how to distribute energy throughout the day to ensure essential activities are completed while avoiding overexertion. Some strategies for effective energy allocation include:

- **Establish a Daily Energy Budget**: Set realistic expectations for daily energy expenditure based on your individual capabilities and limitations. Allocate energy resources to essential tasks while leaving room for rest and relaxation.
- **Plan Ahead**: Anticipate upcoming activities and events and schedule them strategically to coincide with periods of higher energy. Avoid scheduling multiple energy-intensive tasks back-to-back, and allow time for rest and recovery between activities.
- **Use Energy-Saving Techniques**: To conserve energy throughout the day, adopt energy-saving techniques such as pacing your activities, taking regular breaks, and practicing relaxation techniques. Listen to cues from your body and adjust activities accordingly to prevent energy depletion.

- **Flexibility and Adaptability**: Remain flexible and adaptable in managing energy levels, especially during periods of symptom exacerbation or fluctuations in fatigue. Be willing to modify plans or delegate tasks as needed to accommodate changes in energy levels.
- **Monitor and Adjust**: Use a daily log or journal to track energy levels and activity patterns. Look for signs of fatigue or overexertion, and adjust your energy expenditure accordingly. If energy management becomes challenging, seek support from healthcare professionals or support networks.

By implementing these energy conservation strategies, individuals with MG can effectively manage their energy levels, minimize fatigue, and optimize their overall well-being. With careful planning, mindful movement, and task prioritization, you can navigate daily activities with greater ease and confidence, ensuring a balance between productivity and self-care.

❄

ENERGY BUDGETING TOOLS AND TECHNIQUES

Effective energy management for individuals living with MG requires using practical tools and techniques to track energy levels, plan activities strategically, and adjust strategies based on individual needs and patterns. By employing these tools and techniques, you can gain insight into your personal energy patterns, optimize your daily routines, and minimize fatigue and symptom exacerbation.

Keep a Daily Energy Log: Track Energy, Activity, and Symptoms

One of the most valuable tools for energy management is keeping a daily energy log. This log allows you to track your energy levels, activities, and symptoms throughout the day, providing valuable insights into energy expenditure and identifying patterns that may impact your energy levels. This is one of the very first activities I recommend to my clients, and I generally have them keep a log for two weeks to help identify trends in their MG presentation. Here are some practical suggestions for implementing a daily energy log:

- **Choose a Format**: Choose a convenient and easy-to-use format for your energy log, such as a notebook, a digital app, or a spreadsheet on your computer or smartphone.
- **Record Energy Levels**: Rate your energy levels at various times throughout the day using a scale of 1 to 10, with 1 representing extremely low energy and 10 representing extremely high energy. (For a bit of perspective, since I realize it's difficult to put a number on what you feel—at a "1," I feel like a pile of noodles on the floor. At a "10," I feel like climbing a mountain.) Note any fluctuations or changes in energy levels.
- **Document Activities**: Keep track of activities you engage in throughout the day, including both physical and mental tasks. Note the duration and intensity of each activity.
- **Monitor Symptoms**: Record any MG-related symptoms you experience, such as muscle weakness, fatigue, or difficulty with speech or swallowing. Note the severity and duration of each symptom.
- **Review and Reflect**: Review your energy log at the end of each day to identify patterns and trends. Reflect on

activities that may have contributed to changes in energy levels or symptom exacerbation.

Utilize a Weekly Calendar: Plan Activities Strategically

In addition to a daily energy log, a weekly calendar can help you plan activities strategically and allocate energy resources effectively. By scheduling activities in advance and prioritizing tasks based on energy levels, you can optimize your daily routine and minimize overexertion. Here are some practical suggestions for utilizing a weekly calendar:

- **Plan Ahead**: At the beginning of each week, review your commitments and obligations, including work, appointments, and social engagements. Determine which activities are essential and prioritize them accordingly.
- **Identify Peak Energy Times**: Note times of day when your energy levels are typically highest, such as in the morning or after a period of rest. Schedule more demanding tasks or activities during these peak energy times.
- **Space Out Activities**: Avoid scheduling multiple energy-intensive tasks back-to-back. Instead, space out activities throughout the day and allow time for rest and recovery between tasks.
- **Be Realistic**: Consider your energy levels and limitations when planning activities. Avoid overcommitting yourself, and be willing to adjust your schedule as needed to accommodate changes in energy levels or symptoms.
- **Be Flexible**: Remain flexible and adaptable in your scheduling, especially if unexpected events or

fluctuations in energy levels occur. Be prepared to reschedule or delegate tasks as needed to avoid overexertion.

Monitor Patterns and Adjust Strategies Accordingly

Finally, it's essential to monitor patterns in energy levels and symptoms over time and adjust energy management strategies accordingly. By staying vigilant and responsive to changes in energy patterns, you can fine-tune your approach to energy management and optimize your overall well-being. Here are some practical suggestions for monitoring patterns and adjusting strategies:

- **Review Regularly**: Set aside time weekly or monthly to review your energy logs and calendar entries. Look for trends or patterns in energy levels, activities, and symptoms.
- **Identify Triggers**: Pay attention to activities or situations that consistently impact your energy levels or exacerbate symptoms. Identify potential triggers and consider strategies for minimizing their impact.
- **Experiment with Adjustments**: Based on your observations, experiment with adjustments to your routine or energy management strategies. This may include modifying the timing or duration of activities, incorporating more rest breaks, or seeking support from healthcare professionals.
- **Stay Positive and Persistent**: Energy management is an ongoing process that requires patience and perseverance. Stay positive and celebrate small victories along the way, even if progress is gradual.
- **Seek Support**: If you're struggling with energy management, don't hesitate to seek support from

healthcare professionals, support groups, or loved ones. They can offer guidance, encouragement, and practical tips for optimizing your energy levels and quality of life.

By incorporating these energy budgeting tools and techniques into daily life, individuals with MG can gain greater control over their energy levels, minimize fatigue and symptom exacerbation, and enhance their overall quality of life. With dedication and perseverance, energy management can become a valuable tool for living well with MG.

※

MAXIMIZING ENERGY EFFICIENCY THROUGHOUT THE DAY

Strategies for Optimizing High-Energy Times

To make the most of your high-energy times, it's crucial to prioritize tasks that demand the most energy during these periods. Here are some practical strategies for optimizing your high-energy times:

- **Identify Peak Energy Times**: Observe your natural energy patterns and note when you typically feel most energetic during the day. This might be in the morning, after a meal, or after a rest period. Recognizing these peak energy times allows you to schedule important tasks accordingly.
- **Schedule Important Tasks**: Plan to tackle demanding tasks during peak energy times. Allocating work assignments, household chores, or exercise routines to

times when you feel most alert and capable will help you approach tasks with heightened focus and productivity.

- **Break Tasks into Manageable Segments**: Dividing larger tasks into smaller, manageable segments can prevent overwhelm and conserve your energy reserves. Rather than attempting to complete a task all at once, break it down into achievable steps. This approach helps you maintain momentum and progress without draining your energy.

- **Prioritize Activities**: During high-energy times, concentrate on activities aligned with your goals and priorities. Whether pursuing hobbies, spending time with loved ones, or engaging in self-care, use these periods to invest in activities that bring you joy.

Balancing Rest and Activity

Maintaining a balance between rest and activity is essential for managing energy levels effectively and preventing fatigue. Here are some practical strategies for finding equilibrium:

- **Listen to Your Body**: Tune in to your body's signals and recognize when you need rest. If you feel tired or fatigued, take breaks as needed throughout the day, even during high-energy periods. Responding to your body's cues helps prevent exhaustion and conserve energy.

- **Pace Yourself**: Avoid pushing yourself to exhaustion by pacing your activities and incorporating regular rest breaks. Divide tasks into smaller segments and alternate between periods of activity and rest to sustain energy levels. Pacing yourself allows for sustained productivity without burnout.

- **Practice Mindful Rest**: Integrate mindfulness and relaxation techniques into your daily routine to promote rest and relaxation. Dedicate time to activities that help you unwind, such as meditation, deep breathing exercises, or gentle stretching. Mindful rest reduces stress and tension, replenishing your energy reserves.
- **Establish a Bedtime Routine**: Cultivate a relaxing bedtime routine to promote restful sleep and enhance energy levels. Avoid stimulating activities before bed, and create a tranquil sleep environment. Consistent bedtime routines improve sleep quality, ensuring you wake up refreshed and energized.

Incorporate Relaxation Techniques to Recharge

Incorporating relaxation techniques into your daily routine can recharge your energy levels and reduce stress. Here are some effective relaxation techniques to consider:

- **Deep Breathing**: Engage in deep breathing exercises to promote relaxation and alleviate stress. Take slow, deep breaths, inhaling through your nose and exhaling through your mouth. Deep breathing calms the nervous system, reduces stress, and promotes relaxation.
- **Progressive Muscle Relaxation**: Practice progressive muscle relaxation by systematically tensing and releasing muscle groups. Start with your toes and work your way up to your head, focusing on releasing tension. (Note: When tensing muscles during this activity, your effort should be minimal—just enough to turn on the muscle and then relax it. The point of this activity is to get your muscles to relax, not to strengthen or fatigue them.)

- **Meditation**: Incorporate meditation into your routine to quiet the mind and reduce stress. Find a quiet, comfortable space, and focus on your breath or a calming visualization. Meditation fosters mental clarity and relaxation, helping you reduce your stress level while physically relaxing.
- **Guided Imagery**: Use guided imagery to create mental images of peaceful environments. Visualize yourself in serene settings, such as a beach or forest, and immerse yourself in the experience. Guided imagery reduces stress and promotes relaxation.

Low-Energy Rest Activities

In addition to traditional forms of rest like napping, incorporating low-energy rest activities can recharge your energy levels without exerting additional effort. Consider activities such as:

- **Listening to Audiobooks or Podcasts**: Enjoy the immersive experience of listening to audiobooks or podcasts while reclining or resting. Choose topics that interest you and allow your mind to relax and unwind.
- **Gentle Stretching**: Engage in gentle stretching exercises to release tension and promote relaxation. Focus on slow, deliberate movements that encourage flexibility and ease muscle tightness.
- **Mindful Coloring or Drawing**: Embrace the calming effects of coloring or drawing as a restful activity. Use coloring books or sketch pads to express creativity and unwind in a soothing environment.

By implementing these practical strategies for maximizing energy efficiency throughout the day, individuals with MG can better manage their energy levels, minimize fatigue, and optimize their overall well-being. Balancing rest and activity, incorporating relaxation techniques, and integrating low-energy rest activities into daily life foster resilience and promote a balanced approach to energy management.

❄

AVOID ENERGY OVERDRAFT

Living with MG demands a delicate balance between managing energy levels and avoiding burnout. This requires a deep understanding of one's body and its signals, as well as proactive strategies to prevent overexertion. By recognizing the signs of energy depletion and implementing practical techniques for energy conservation, individuals with MG can navigate their daily lives more effectively while preserving their overall quality of life.

Just as you don't want to overdraw your bank account, don't overdraw your energy store.

Recognize Signs of Energy Depletion and Overexertion

Recognizing signs of energy depletion and overexertion is central to managing energy levels with MG. Signs of energy depletion may vary from person to person but commonly include:

- **Muscle Weakness**: Increased difficulty performing previously manageable tasks may indicate depletion of energy reserves, particularly in muscles affected by MG fatigable weakness.
- **Fatigue**: Persistent feelings of exhaustion, even after

adequate rest, can indicate that the body's energy stores are nearing depletion.

- **Increased Symptoms**: A worsening of MG symptoms, such as drooping eyelids, double vision, or difficulty speaking or swallowing, may signal overexertion and the need for rest.
- **Mental Fog**: Difficulty concentrating, cognitive fog, or memory lapses can occur when the brain is fatigued and overwhelmed by excessive energy expenditure.
- **Emotional Changes**: Irritability, mood swings, or feelings of frustration and overwhelm may indicate that you are pushing yourself beyond your limits and experiencing emotional fatigue.

Being attuned to your body's signals is crucial in identifying when you're nearing your energy limits. To help conceptualize these signs, consider using a stoplight analogy:

- **Green Light**: Indicates that all is well and you are operating within your energy limits.
- **Yellow Light**: Serves as a cautionary signal where signs of fatigue appear. It's essential to slow down and rest to prevent further depletion of energy reserves.
- **Red Light**: Indicates a severe worsening of symptoms that should be a <u>hard stop</u> for activity. The critical difference between yellow and red in this analogy is that at yellow, you still have the choice of whether or not to continue an activity. At red, your body will stop you, and *this is a potentially dangerous place to be.*

Set Realistic Goals and Limits

Setting realistic goals and limits is essential for managing energy levels effectively and preventing flare-ups and exacerbations. By establishing clear boundaries and prioritizing self-care, you can maintain a healthy balance between activity and rest. Practical strategies for setting realistic goals and limits include:

- **Prioritize Tasks**: Identify and prioritize essential tasks based on importance and urgency. Focus on completing high-priority tasks during periods of higher energy while allowing less critical tasks to wait or be delegated to others.
- **Break Tasks into Manageable Steps**: Breaking larger tasks into smaller, more manageable steps can prevent overwhelm and conserve energy. Setting achievable goals for each step can also maintain motivation and avoid burnout.
- **Know Your Limits**: It's crucial to be realistic about your energy levels and recognize when to scale back or take breaks. Listening to your body's cues and honoring your limits is essential for preventing overexertion and maintaining overall well-being.
- **Set Boundaries**: Learn to say "no" to additional commitments or requests that may strain your energy resources. Setting boundaries around your time and energy allows you to prioritize activities that support your physical and mental health.
- **Be Flexible**: Flexibility is vital when managing energy levels with MG. Being willing to adjust goals and plans based on changes in energy levels or symptoms enables you to adapt to your body's needs and prevent flare-ups.

Practice Self-Care and Listen to Your Body

Incorporating self-care practices into daily life is crucial for managing energy levels and preventing burnout. Prioritizing rest, healthy habits, and stress management can help individuals living with MG maintain a sustainable energy level while enhancing resilience. Self-care practices to consider include:

- **Rest and Relaxation**: Making time for rest and relaxation each day is essential for recharging energy levels. Engaging in activities that promote relaxation, such as reading, listening to music, or practicing mindfulness, can help you unwind and replenish your energy reserves.
- **Healthy Habits**: Maintaining a healthy lifestyle through proper nutrition, hydration, and gentle exercise within energy limits is essential for supporting your overall well-being. Prioritizing activities that promote physical and mental health can help you maintain your energy levels and prevent burnout.
- **Stress Management**: Stress-reduction techniques, such as meditation, deep breathing exercises, or progressive muscle relaxation, can help you manage stress and promote relaxation. Incorporating these techniques into daily life can help you cope more effectively with the challenges of MG.
- **Social Support**: Seeking support from friends, family, or support groups can provide valuable encouragement and assistance when managing energy levels with MG. Connecting with others who understand your condition can help you feel supported and less isolated.
- **Professional Help**: Seeking guidance from healthcare professionals, such as doctors or therapists, can provide

additional support and resources for managing energy levels with MG. Healthcare professionals can offer personalized advice, treatment options, and support tailored to your individual needs.

By recognizing signs of energy depletion, setting realistic goals and limits, and prioritizing self-care, individuals living with MG can minimize the risk of exacerbation and maintain a balanced approach to managing their energy levels. Taking proactive steps to protect and preserve energy resources is essential for optimizing overall well-being and quality of life with MG.

❄

To effectively manage energy levels with MG, it's crucial to adopt the concept of energy budgeting, which is similar to managing finances. Just as you allocate money for different expenses, recognizing and living within your energy budget entails allocating energy for various activities throughout the day. Understanding your body's signals and establishing energy limits is critical. Signs of depletion or overexertion, like muscle weakness and increased symptoms, serve as indicators to avoid pushing beyond your limits. Prioritizing self-care through practices such as rest, nutrition, and stress management is essential to conserve energy and promote resilience. Additionally, remaining adaptable and flexible with plans and activities based on energy levels and symptoms allows for smoother navigation of daily life with MG. By embracing energy budgeting and prioritizing self-care, you can effectively manage your energy levels and enhance your overall quality of life.

ACTION ITEMS

1. **Create an Energy Budget**: Keep a daily log of your energy levels, activity levels, and symptom progression. This will help you identify patterns and understand how different activities impact your energy reserves. Use this information to create an energy budget, allocating your energy resources wisely throughout the day and prioritizing activities during periods of higher energy.

2. **Set Realistic Goals and Boundaries**: Identify your priorities and set realistic goals based on your energy levels and limitations. Break tasks into manageable steps, and prioritize self-care to prevent overexertion and burnout. Practice saying "no" to additional commitments or requests that may strain your energy resources, and be willing to adjust your goals and plans as needed based on changes in your energy levels or symptoms.

3. **Practice Self-Care and Listen to Your Body**: Incorporate self-care practices into your daily routine to support your physical and mental well-being. Make time for rest and relaxation, eat nutritious foods, stay hydrated, and engage in gentle exercise within your energy limits. Listen to your body's cues, and honor your limits, seeking support from healthcare professionals or loved ones when needed.

BONUS! Need a few templates and guides to help you create your energy budget? Good news! I've got templates for a daily energy and activity log, a pacing calendar, and more! Download the supplemental resource pack at www.lizplowman.com/spoons.

Chapter 3

Assistive Devices

Generalized Myasthenia Gravis (GMG) causes muscle fatigue and weakness that can affect mobility. Assistive devices, such as canes, walkers, crutches, etc., do precisely that: *assist*. The right assistive device can go a long way toward helping you with mobility and energy conservation.

Here are five signs that it might be time to consider an assistive device:

1. **You are wobbly on your feet**. Even if you aren't losing your balance or falling, simply feeling "wobbly" or unsteady is an early sign that the stabilizing muscles in your legs need a little help.
2. **You "furniture surf."** If you frequently walk with the help of the walls, the back of the sofa, etc., then your body is already telling you that it needs some help to get around safely.
3. **You have trouble walking through the grocery store**. If you are fatigued by prolonged periods of walking and standing (like in the grocery store), an assistive device can

help you conserve energy so that you can stand and walk longer before fatiguing.

4. **You shuffle or drag your feet**. This is a sign that your hip flexors (the muscles that lift your leg and advance it forward while walking) are weak and fatigued. This increases the risk of stumbling and falling.

5. **You stumble, lose your balance, or fall**. If you are already losing balance or even falling, then it's definitely time to consider an assistive device to keep you safe and prevent injury.

If you notice any of these signs, it's probably time to start using an assistive device to conserve your energy, prevent falls, and improve your mobility. If you'd like help selecting the best device and learning how to use it, keep reading!

❄

Personal Vignette: The First Time I Used a Cane

I was standing at the edge of the park, a simple cane in my hand for the first time, feeling the burden of weakness and fatigue pulling at my muscles. Thanks, MG... But for a moment, as I looked out at the vibrant green grass and heard my one-year-old daughter's voice calling me to join her, I felt something unfamiliar: hope.

"Ma-ma?" she asked, her little hand beckoning me forward. Of course I was. I gripped my cane tighter and took a deep breath, determined not to let this disease hold me back.

As I walked with my husband by my side, I thought back to our early morning runs—the times I would drag him out of bed at the crack of dawn to run by the water or on a chilly woodland trail. Those days seemed like a distant memory now that my legs were weak and fatigued. Again, thank you, MG...

But with my trusty new cane tapping against the ground, I could feel a newfound sense of confidence and freedom. "Let's see how far we can get today," my husband encouraged me.

And so we walked, slowly at first, but then picking up speed as my heart swelled with joy. It was just a casual family outing, but it felt like so much more. My daughter toddled ahead without a care in the world while I reveled in the simple pleasure of being able to move again.

"Mommy's coming," I said under my breath, feeling grateful for this small victory over my illness. This simple bright blue aluminum cane that I had picked up at the pharmacy—my reluctant ally—had become my wings, giving me the courage to embrace change and accept help.

As we caught up to our daughter and she saw me walking towards her, her face lit up with excitement and love. In that moment, I realized that strength doesn't always look like what we expect it to. Sometimes, it looks like accepting help and pushing through obstacles with the unwavering support of loved ones by our side. With my cane as my ally and my family as my rock, I knew I could face whatever challenges lay ahead.

This was a pivotal moment in my personal journey with MG—a moment that echoes the uncertainty and reluctance many of us feel when faced with the prospect of using assistive devices.

Despite the daily challenges posed by MG, I was hesitant to embrace the idea of relying on an assistive device. Thoughts swirled in my mind: "I'm young and otherwise healthy—what will people think if they see me with a cane or a walker?" It felt like a visible admission of vulnerability, and I grappled with the fear of judgment.

But life has a way of nudging us towards necessary realizations. The turning point came when the desire to actively participate in outdoor activities with my family—activities that had slowly slipped away—outweighed the fear of any perceived judgments. With a mixture of trepidation and determination, I decided to give a simple cane a try.

The initial steps were met with internal resistance as if the device symbolized a concession to my condition. However, as I leaned on that cane, a subtle transformation occurred. Instead of weakness, I felt a newfound strength in every step. The support it provided became a bridge between the limitations imposed by MG and the life I yearned to lead.

As the days, weeks, and months unfolded, I found myself exploring other assistive devices—each step a calculated response to the evolving nature of my condition at that time. From a cane to forearm crutches to eventually a power wheelchair, each device became a gateway to experiences that once seemed distant. The joy of strolling through a park, the laughter during a family outing, taking my kids trick-or-treating at Halloween, and the freedom to engage in activities without the constant weight of fatigue—these moments became a testament to the liberating power of assistive devices.

Navigating the world with a mobility aid was not about succumbing to weakness but a strategic move toward empowerment. It wasn't just about what people might think; it was about what I could achieve, the memories I could create, and the life I could continue to lead despite MG.

Choosing to use an assistive device was not a surrender; it was a declaration of resilience. It opened doors to a world of possibilities that I hadn't envisioned. The once-reluctant steps with a cane paved the way for a journey filled with newfound independence and the ability to cherish moments with my family.

As you consider incorporating assistive devices into your life, know you are not alone in your hesitation. Your journey is uniquely yours, and the decision to use these tools is not a reflection of weakness but a testament to your strength, adaptability, and unwavering spirit that propels us forward.

❄

RECOGNIZING THE NEED FOR AN ASSISTIVE DEVICE

Deciding when to use an assistive device is a personal decision that requires self-awareness and understanding of your MG symptoms. Here are some signs that you might need additional support:

- **Persistent Weakness:** If muscle weakness frequently affects your mobility or daily activities, it may be time to consider an assistive device. Continuous muscle weakness can impact your overall well-being, so finding ways to improve stability and movement is essential.
- **Chronic Fatigue:** Chronic fatigue is a common symptom of MG and can make it challenging to sustain physical activity. If fatigue constantly affects your energy levels and daily tasks, an assistive device could help reduce physical strain and conserve energy for essential activities.
- **Difficulty Walking:** If walking becomes challenging due to muscle weakness or imbalance, it may be a clear sign that you need extra support. Assistive devices can provide the stability and balance required to move confidently and reduce the risk of falls.

Recognizing these signs allows you to make informed decisions about using assistive devices. By acknowledging the need for extra support, you take a proactive step to improve your quality of life and better manage your journey with MG.

❄

CHOOSING THE RIGHT ASSISTIVE DEVICE

Choosing the right assistive device is an essential step in effectively managing MG. Each device has benefits and potential drawbacks, which you should consider when selecting the best one for you. By understanding the features and functions of these devices, you can make informed decisions that suit your specific needs and preferences and select the best tools to enhance your quality of life and maintain your independence.

Canes:

- **Benefits:** Canes offer stability and balance support with a simple, lightweight design. They are easy to use and portable, making them a convenient choice for daily activities. Canes are relatively inexpensive and easy to obtain compared with other assistive devices.
- **Drawbacks:** Canes may be limited in providing extensive weight-bearing assistance. In cases of severe weakness, a cane might not offer the robust support required to navigate certain activities or terrains.

Walkers:

- **Benefits:** Walkers present an enhanced level of stability with a broader base of support. Some models even come equipped with seats, providing a convenient option for resting during longer excursions. Walkers can be particularly helpful for people with extensive hip flexor weakness (difficulty lifting the leg or advancing it forward when walking).

- **Drawbacks:** Walkers can be bulky and challenging to maneuver in tight or crowded spaces. Due to their size and weight, transporting and storing them can be cumbersome. Additionally, users may find them less discreet than more compact devices.

PRO TIP: *Use the "shopping cart test." If you have an easier time walking when pushing a shopping cart, you may do well with a walker.*

Crutches:

- **Benefits:** Crutches distribute weight effectively across the upper body, providing substantial support for both legs. They help maintain balance and facilitate movement, particularly for those with hip extensor or gluteal weakness (difficulty standing upright or pushing your body forward when walking).
- **Drawbacks:** Crutches require significant upper body strength for effective use. Extended use can be tiring, particularly for individuals dealing with upper body fatigue associated with MG. Crutches may also limit the ability to carry items while moving.

Manual Wheelchairs:

- **Benefits:** Manual wheelchairs offer full mobility without requiring leg strength. They are self-propelled, so they never need to be recharged. Most manual wheelchairs can collapse down to fit in the trunk or backseat of a car.
- **Drawbacks:** Manual wheelchair use relies predominantly on arm strength, which can be

challenging for those with upper body muscle weakness and fatigue. Negotiating uphill terrain may pose a challenge, potentially requiring assistance. Like a walker, manual wheelchairs can be bulky and cumbersome and may not do well in tight or crowded spaces. They can also be challenging to transport and store.

Power Wheelchairs:

- **Benefits:** Power wheelchairs provide greater independence through electric propulsion. They are well-suited for extended use and offer a practical solution for those seeking efficient mobility. They are easy to maneuver with minimal physical effort, making them ideal for people with severe muscle weakness.
- **Drawbacks:** Power wheelchairs are significantly heavier and bulkier than their manual counterparts. They are incredibly cumbersome to transport, requiring a trailer, wheelchair-accessible vehicle, or reliable access to accessible public transportation. They require regular maintenance, including frequently charging the batteries. The initial cost and potential repair expenses can be higher compared to manual wheelchairs, and they may not be a financially viable option with significant insurance assistance.

Electric Scooters:

- **Benefits:** Electric scooters allow independence through electric propulsion like a power wheelchair but are a less bulky, more portable, and less expensive option. They provide a comfortable and efficient means of transportation, catering to individuals seeking a versatile travel solution. Electric scooters are often available to borrow or rent from venues such as grocery stores, large museums, and amusement parks for use while on the premises.

- **Drawbacks:** Their utility may be limited to specific terrains, as they might struggle on rough or uneven surfaces. Electric scooters are bulkier than canes or walkers, affecting ease of use and storage. While transporting a scooter is slightly more manageable than a power wheelchair, you will still need a capable vehicle or accessible public transportation options. Regular maintenance and battery charging are necessary to ensure consistent performance. Lastly, scooters require more upper body strength and endurance than power wheelchairs because they have a handlebar-style steering set-up. Some people with MG may find that this fatigues their shoulders quickly.

Consider your unique needs, lifestyle, and preferences when navigating this diverse landscape of assistive devices. Each device has its advantages and considerations, and the key is finding the one that seamlessly integrates into your life, empowering you to navigate the challenges MG poses with confidence and independence.

❄

FITTING YOUR ASSISTIVE DEVICE

Selecting the right assistive device is only the first step. Ensuring a proper fit is equally crucial to maximize its effectiveness and promote your overall comfort. Whether it's a cane, crutches, walker, or wheelchair, the right fit enhances stability, reduces strain, and minimizes the risk of potential discomfort. (Side note: As a physical therapist, I can't begin to tell you how much it irks me to see people using assistive devices that are not correctly fit!)

Consider the following guidelines for proper fit and use of your assistive device. If you need additional guidance, seek out a physical therapist for help.

Canes:

- **Height Adjustment:** Adjust the cane's height so that the top of the handle aligns with your wrist crease when your arms hang comfortably at your sides.
- **Grip Comfort:** Choose a cane with a comfortable grip. When holding the cane, your elbow should be slightly bent at about 30 degrees, allowing for a natural and efficient posture.
- **Wrist Position:** Ensure your wrist does not hyperextend when gripping the cane. A neutral wrist position optimizes grip stability and minimizes wrist joint strain during use.

Walkers:

- **Height Adjustment:** Adjust the walker's height so that the handles are at the level of your wrist crease when your arms hang naturally.
- **Grip Comfort:** Similar to canes, choose a walker with comfortable grips. When holding the handles, your elbows should be comfortably bent at a 30-degree angle.
- **Width:** The walker frame should be wide enough to stand inside of comfortably. If the walker is too narrow, you'll have to position it too far in front of your body,

diminishing its ability to support you and potentially increasing your risk of fall and injury. (I realize this may be a touchy subject for some, but please consider a bariatric walker if frame width is a concern. Function and safety are paramount, so be sure to select a walker frame that is wide enough to allow for proper use.)

Axillary (Traditional) Crutches:

- **Height Adjustment:** Adjust the crutches' height so that the top of the crutch pad is about 1-2 inches below your armpits. Many crutches have a height guide printed on the frame, which is a helpful place to start, but please keep in mind that this is a rough guideline only. Also, remember that you may need to adjust the crutches up or down depending on your shoe height.
- **Handgrip Position:** Position the handgrips at a comfortable level, allowing for a 30-degree bend in your elbows when standing. This prevents wrist strain and promotes proper weight distribution.

Forearm (Lofstrand) Crutches:

- **Height Adjustment:** Set the height of the forearm crutches so that the top of the cuffs sit 1-1.5 inches below your elbows when your arms hang naturally. As with the height guidelines for axillary crutches above, only use the pre-printed height markings as a rough guide.
- **Forearm Cuff Position:** Position the forearm cuffs to provide support without pressing into your forearms. Your hands should comfortably grip the handgrips, allowing for a 30-degree elbow bend.

- **Handgrip Angle:** Adjust the handgrip angle to align with your natural wrist position, avoiding hyperextension.

Wheelchairs:

[NOTE: Not all wheelchairs are adjustable, particularly "off the shelf" models. If you have the ability to get a custom wheelchair, your vendor should take measurements and ensure a correct fit. If your wheelchair is not adjustable, consider the following guidelines to determine if your wheelchair is a good model for your body type.]

- **Seat Height:** When seated, your knees should be at a 90-degree angle. If possible, adjust the seat height and/or footrests or footplate (depending on the model) so that your feet rest comfortably on them.
- **Armrest Height:** Set the armrests at a height that allows your shoulders to relax and your elbows to bend comfortably at a 90-degree angle.
- **Wheelchair Width:** Ensure the wheelchair's width accommodates your hips comfortably without causing pressure points.

Remember, these fitting guidelines serve as a general reference. Individual variations may apply, so it's advisable to consult with a physical therapist to fine-tune the fit of your chosen assistive device. A well-fitted device enhances its functionality and contributes to your overall well-being as you navigate life with MG.

❄

Dr. Liz Plowman

TIPS FOR EFFECTIVE USE

Proper training is paramount when incorporating an assistive device into your routine. Seek guidance from a physical therapist to learn the correct usage and techniques tailored to your specific needs. They can provide valuable insights on optimizing the benefits of your chosen device and ensuring your safety during daily activities.

Gradual integration is a key strategy to facilitate a smooth adjustment period. Rather than diving headfirst into using the device extensively, start by incorporating it into select activities. This approach allows your body to adapt gradually, building both physical and mental comfort with the new support system.

Regular maintenance is essential to guarantee the continued reliability of your assistive device. Like any tool, these devices require upkeep to function at their best. Establish a routine for checking and maintaining your device, promptly addressing any wear and tear. This proactive approach ensures that your device remains a dependable ally in navigating the challenges posed by MG.

❄

ADAPTING TO YOUR ENERGY LEVEL: SWITCHING BETWEEN ASSISTIVE DEVICES

Navigating life with MG often involves a dynamic interplay of energy levels, fatigue, and the ever-changing landscape of daily activities. Energy levels are frequently a moving target that changes day to day (or hour to hour). Being able to transition between different assistive devices depending on your energy level and weakness pattern is a skill that empowers individuals with MG to optimize their energy conservation based on their needs at any given time.

Listen to Your Body

Understanding your body's cues is the cornerstone of effective device management. Pay attention to fluctuations in energy levels and muscle strength throughout the day. When fatigue sets in or when you need extra support, select a more supportive assistive device.

Match Devices to Activities

Different activities call for varying levels of support. For short, brisk walks, a cane provides enough stability without being cumbersome. More extended outings might necessitate using a walker or even a wheelchair to conserve energy. Assessing the demands of each activity allows you to select the most appropriate device, optimizing both comfort and efficiency.

Strategic Device Transitions

Switching between devices strategically can be a game-changer. For example, beginning your day with a cane for morning mobility might preserve energy for later tasks. As fatigue sets in, transitioning to a walker or wheelchair for more extended excursions ensures continued participation without compromising safety or well-being.

Adapt to Your Environment

Consider the specific challenges presented by different environments. Tight spaces may favor a cane or forearm crutches, whereas a wheelchair could offer greater safety and stability in crowded areas, reducing the risk that someone may bump into you and cause you to fall. Large areas that require navigating long distances, such as a shopping center or an amusement park, may be better served by an electric scooter or power wheelchair. Adapting your choice of device to the environment enhances your ability to navigate seamlessly and comfortably.

Effective Communication

Open communication with those around you is instrumental in creating a supportive environment. When you communicate your energy levels and device preferences, friends, family, and colleagues can better understand your needs. This strengthens your support network and alleviates any potential discomfort or misconceptions.

Building Confidence

Switching between assistive devices is not a sign of inconsistency or weakness; it's a testament to your adaptability and resilience. Embracing this versatility builds confidence in your ability to navigate the ebb and flow of MG symptoms. It allows you to actively participate in a broad spectrum of activities, contributing to a more fulfilling and empowered lifestyle.

In the dynamic dance of MG management, the ability to switch between assistive devices is a valuable skill. It's not just about adapting to physical challenges but also about crafting a lifestyle that revolves around your energy levels and individual needs. By mastering the art of transitioning between devices, you can reclaim control over your daily experiences and pave the way for a more empowered and adaptable journey with MG.

❄

ADDRESSING EMOTIONAL CHALLENGES

Embracing independence is not just a physical adjustment but also a mindset shift. Focus on the newfound freedom and empowerment that these devices provide. Recognize them as tools that amplify your capabilities, enabling you to engage in activities and experiences that bring joy and fulfillment. The ability to move with greater ease is not a sign of limitation but a pathway to liberation.

Open communication is crucial in navigating the emotional aspects of using assistive devices. Share your thoughts and concerns with friends, family, and healthcare professionals. Discussing your journey openly fosters understanding and support from those around you. It allows you to dispel any misconceptions, build a robust support system, and reinforce the idea that using these devices is a proactive decision to enhance your overall well-being.

Remember, the journey with MG is not just a physical one—it's a whole human experience that encompasses your emotional and mental well-being, too. Addressing the practical and emotional aspects of incorporating assistive devices can pave the way for a more enriching and fulfilling life.

As we conclude this chapter on assistive devices, remember that living with MG is a personal journey marked by unique challenges and triumphs. Embracing assistive devices is a strategic move towards empowerment, not a surrender to weakness. The devices discussed here are allies in your quest for a fulfilling and active life. From canes to walkers, crutches to wheelchairs, and the strategic art of switching between them, each choice reflects your resilience and adaptability. As you manage energy conservation and device use, may you find control, flexibility, and confidence, leading to a life filled with possibilities and joy.

Chapter 4

Life Hacks

LIVING WITH MYASTHENIA GRAVIS (MG) CAN PRESENT many challenges and obstacles in daily life. From fatigue and weakness to difficulty with mobility and fine motor skills, the symptoms of MG can make even the simplest tasks seem daunting. As a physical therapist, I am trained, among other things, to help people optimize their physical functionality. With MG though, the rules are different. It isn't only about not pushing your physical boundaries but also about knowing when to conserve your energy and pace yourself. This involves a delicate and constant dance between doing what you can and acknowledging what you need help with. With some practical and creative life hacks, you can make life with MG easier, more productive, and more comfortable.

In this chapter, we will explore various aspects of your home and personal care, such as the bathroom, the kitchen, the work area, the car, and household chores, and suggest modifications, adaptations, and shortcuts that can help conserve physical energy and avoid unnecessary strain or stress on the body.

❄

Bathroom Hacks

- **Install grab bars:** Weakness in the arms and legs can pose a significant challenge when navigating the bathroom. To enhance safety and ease of movement, strategically install sturdy grab bars. Place them in and near the bathtub or shower, around the toilet, and along the walls as needed for additional support. Opt for grab bars with a non-slip surface to ensure a secure grip. These bars provide stability and reduce the risk of slips and falls, offering a helping hand when you need it most. While removable suction cup grab bars are an option for smooth surfaces (e.g., shower walls), they are far less secure than permanently installed bars. Use these with caution!

- **Use a shower chair:** Long periods of standing can be particularly draining for individuals with MG. Transform your shower routine by incorporating a shower chair. This simple addition allows you to sit and relax while showering, conserving energy for other activities. Look for a chair with a comfortable seat, a backrest, and non-slip feet to ensure a secure and comfortable experience. With a shower chair, you can turn your shower time into a rejuvenating break without worrying about fatigue.

- **Use a raised toilet seat:** Weakness in the legs can make rising from a low toilet seat a challenging task. Upgrade your bathroom with a raised toilet seat to alleviate this obstacle. These seats fit securely on top of the existing toilet, providing a higher surface for easier standing. Look for models with sturdy handles for added support. A raised toilet seat can be a game-changer, promoting independence and reducing the physical strain associated with using standard toilet facilities.

- **Install a handheld shower head:** Enhance your shower experience by installing a handheld shower head. This modification allows you to control the direction and flow of water while seated, offering flexibility and convenience. With a handheld shower head, you can target specific areas without unnecessary movements. It also allows you to perform your bathing activities while sitting rather than frequently standing to rinse off. Choose a model with an easy-to-reach holder, ensuring the shower head is always within your grasp. This small change can make a big difference in conserving energy during your daily hygiene routine.

- **Use non-slip mats and rugs:** The bathroom floor can be a potential hazard, especially for those with balance issues. Invest in non-slip mats or rugs to enhance stability and reduce the risk of slipping. Place these mats strategically near the shower, bathtub, and sink areas. Opt for designs that have a low profile and are highly visible to reduce the risk of tripping and potentially falling. Non-slip mats provide a secure footing, adding an extra layer of safety to your bathroom environment.

- **Consider a walk-in bathtub or shower:** Traditional bathtubs can be challenging to navigate for individuals with mobility issues. Explore the option of a walk-in bathtub or shower for added convenience. These designs feature a low threshold, allowing for easier entry and exit. With walk-in options, you can maintain your independence and enjoy a soothing bath or shower without the stress of climbing over high edges.

- **Organize with baskets and caddies:** Simplify your bathroom routine by organizing your essentials with baskets and caddies. Keep frequently used items neatly arranged and easily accessible. Use baskets to store towels, toiletries, and other necessities. Caddies can hold shower products and keep them within arm's reach. By creating an organized space with easy access to your frequently used items, you conserve energy and streamline your daily routine.

- **Consider adaptive grooming tools:** Explore grooming tools designed with adaptability in mind. Look for lightweight and ergonomic hairbrushes, razors, and other grooming essentials that reduce strain on your hands and arms. Consider a mounted hair dryer stand to reduce arm strain when styling your hair. Adaptive tools often feature larger handles for a better grip, making them more accessible and comfortable for individuals with muscle weakness.

- **Optimize toweling techniques:** Drying off after a shower or bath can be physically demanding. Consider optimizing your toweling techniques to conserve energy. Instead of vigorous rubbing, gently pat your skin with a soft and absorbent towel. Invest in quick-drying towels to reduce the time spent on this task. Additionally, consider using a bathrobe or a towel wrap to absorb excess water and minimize the effort required for toweling off, especially if muscle weakness affects your range of motion.

- **Sit whenever you can:** Applying makeup, shaving, or performing other grooming tasks while seated can be more comfortable and energy-efficient. Instead of standing at the sink or in front of the mirror, conveniently place a chair or stool to allow you to sit for tasks like brushing your hair or applying products.

Remember, these bathroom hacks are adaptable to your unique needs and preferences. Feel free to explore different modifications and discover the combination that best enhances your comfort and convenience in the bathroom.

Kitchen Hacks

- **Use kitchen gadgets:** Embrace the power of kitchen gadgets designed to simplify food preparation. Jar openers, electric can openers, and food processors can be invaluable tools for individuals with MG. Invest in these gadgets to save both time and energy in the kitchen. Electric can openers, in particular, eliminate the need for manual twisting, making the process effortless. Similarly, food processors can easily handle chopping and slicing tasks, reducing the strain on your hands and wrists.
- **Sit while cooking:** Transform your cooking routine by incorporating a seating option. Whether using a stool or a comfortable chair, sitting while cooking can significantly conserve your energy. Position your seat near the countertop or stove to maintain easy access to your workspace. This simple adjustment reduces fatigue and allows you to enjoy the creative process of cooking without the physical strain of prolonged standing.
- **Use lightweight cookware:** Heavy pots and pans can pose a challenge, especially for those with significant arm muscle weakness. Upgrade your cookware to lightweight alternatives to ease the lifting and maneuvering process. Opt for materials like aluminum or non-stick coatings, which are easier to handle and simplify the cleaning process. Lightweight cookware ensures that preparing

meals remains a joyous activity without unnecessary physical strain.

- **Utilize a rolling cart or trolley:** When transporting dishes, pots, and pans around the kitchen, introduce the convenience of a rolling cart or trolley. This smart solution eliminates the need to carry heavy items, reducing strain on your arms and minimizing fatigue. Choose a sturdy cart with wheels that can easily navigate your kitchen floor. This way, you can effortlessly transfer items from one station to another without exerting undue effort.

- **Invest in one-handed kitchen tools:** Explore kitchen tools designed for one-handed use, providing enhanced accessibility for individuals with limited strength or coordination. Look for utensils, cutting boards, and peelers intended to be operated with a single hand. These specialized tools make cooking more feasible and empower you to enjoy a greater level of independence in the kitchen. From one-handed can openers to adaptive knives, there's a variety of tools tailored to your specific needs.

- **Prep ingredients in advance:** Prepping ingredients in advance can save time and energy. Consider chopping vegetables, marinating meats, or measuring ingredients ahead of time. Store these prepped items in labeled containers for easy access during cooking. Prepping in advance streamlines the cooking process, allows you to conserve energy, and allows you to enjoy a more relaxed culinary experience.

- **Embrace convenience with ready-to-use items:** Simplify meal preparation by incorporating ready-to-use items into your kitchen routine. Choose pre-cut vegetables, pre-washed greens, and other convenience products that reduce the need for extensive chopping and washing. While fresh ingredients are lovely, ready-to-use items can be a practical alternative, allowing you to enjoy delicious and nutritious meals without compromising on convenience.

- **Opt for ergonomic kitchen tools:** Choose kitchen tools with ergonomic designs that prioritize comfort and ease of use. Ergonomic utensils, peelers, and cutting tools are crafted to reduce strain on your hands and wrists. Look for options with padded grips and handles that fit comfortably in your hand. These tools enhance your control and efficiency in the kitchen, making daily cooking tasks more manageable and enjoyable.
- **Explore adaptive cutting boards:** Cutting ingredients can be challenging for those with MG. Adaptive cutting boards are designed to provide stability and support during food preparation. Look for boards with non-slip bases and pronged spikes to secure fruits and vegetables in place. Adaptive cutting boards minimize the effort required to chop and slice, allowing you to maintain your culinary creativity with greater ease.

By incorporating these kitchen hacks into your daily routine, you can create a culinary space that aligns with your needs and enhances your cooking experience. Experiment with different strategies to find the combination that suits you best, allowing you to savor the joys of preparing meals without unnecessary physical strain.

Work Area Hacks

- **Invest in an ergonomic chair with head and trunk support:** Transform your work area into a comfortable and supportive space by investing in an ergonomic chair. Look for a chair with adjustable head and trunk support to maintain proper alignment and reduce strain on your neck and back. Adjustable features allow you to customize the chair to your specific needs, promoting a healthy posture during extended work sessions.

- **Utilize voice-to-text software:** Minimize the strain on your hands and fingers during typing tasks by incorporating voice-to-text software. This technology allows you to dictate your thoughts, emails, or documents, reducing the physical demand on your muscles. Explore various voice recognition tools that seamlessly convert your spoken words into written text, enhancing both efficiency and accessibility in your work environment.

- **Optimize screen brightness and contrast:** Combat eye strain and accommodate double vision by optimizing your computer screen's brightness and contrast settings. Adjust these settings to find a balance that reduces glare and enhances visual clarity. Consider using a matte screen filter to further reduce glare. Taking proactive measures to create a visually comfortable environment can significantly improve your ability to focus and work with ease.

- **Use task lighting with adjustable intensity:** Illuminate your workspace with task lighting featuring adjustable intensity settings. This allows you to control the brightness based on your specific needs and preferences. Adequate lighting not only reduces eye strain but also enhances overall visibility. Position the lighting source to minimize shadows and create a well-lit environment that supports your concentration and reduces visual fatigue.

- **Implement the 20-20-20 rule:** Combat eye strain and refresh your eyes by following the 20-20-20 rule. Every 20 minutes, take a 20-second break and focus on something 20 feet away. This simple practice helps reduce eye fatigue caused by prolonged screen exposure. Set reminders or use productivity apps to prompt you to take these short breaks, contributing to long-term eye health.
- **Customize your keyboard and mouse:** Tailor your keyboard and mouse to suit your specific needs. Choose ergonomic designs that minimize strain on your hands and wrists. Consider keyboards with larger keys or special layouts that facilitate easier typing. Similarly, opt for a mouse that fits comfortably in your hand, reducing the risk of repetitive strain injuries. Also, consider supporting your elbows and forearms with a pillow or rolled-up towel in your lap to reduce shoulder fatigue caused by prolonged arm positioning when using a keyboard and mouse.
- **Utilize a document holder:** If you frequently reference documents while working on your computer, use a document holder to position them at eye level. This minimizes the need to constantly shift your gaze between the document and the screen, reducing eye strain and neck discomfort. Adjustable document holders allow you to find the optimal viewing angle, promoting a more ergonomic and comfortable workspace.
- **Explore alternative input devices:** For tasks that involve precise movements or detailed work, explore alternative input devices such as trackballs, touchpads, or stylus pens. These devices can offer a more comfortable and controlled interface, reducing the strain on your hands and fingers. Experiment with different options to

find the input device that best suits your needs and enhances your efficiency.

- **Schedule regular breaks for stretching and movement:** Combat the physical toll of prolonged sitting by scheduling regular breaks for stretching and movement. Incorporate simple stretches or short walks into your routine to promote circulation and reduce muscle stiffness. Set reminders to encourage these breaks, ensuring you maintain a healthy balance between focused work and physical activity throughout the day.
- **Personalize your workspace for motivation:** Create a personalized and motivating workspace by adding elements that bring you joy and inspiration. Decorate your work area with items that evoke positive feelings, whether it's photos, artwork, or meaningful quotes. A visually pleasing and uplifting environment can contribute to a positive mindset, fostering productivity and overall well-being. While I realize this isn't an energy conservation tip, *per se*, a positive environment can go a long way to reducing your stress level, which is helpful in MG.

By incorporating these life hacks into your work area, you can create a workspace that caters to the unique challenges presented by MG. Experiment with different strategies to find the combination that best supports your comfort, productivity, and overall job satisfaction.

Car Hacks

- **Get a handicapped parking permit:** If walking long distances poses a challenge, obtaining a handicapped parking permit can significantly improve your mobility.

This permit allows you to park in designated accessible spaces, reducing the distance you need to travel from your car to your destination. Ensure that you meet the criteria for eligibility and apply for a permit to enhance convenience and conserve your energy for the activities that matter most. While requirements and procedures differ depending on where you live, your physician's office is a great place to start.

- **Use a steering wheel cover:** Combat hand fatigue during extended drives by investing in a quality steering wheel cover. Opt for a cover with a textured surface that provides a comfortable and secure grip. This simple addition reduces strain on your hands and enhances your overall driving experience. Choose materials that are easy to clean and maintain for added convenience.

- **Swivel seat for easy entry and exit:** Installing a swivel seat makes getting in and out of your car a breeze. These seats rotate to face the door, facilitating smoother entry and exit. Swivel seats come in various designs and can be adapted to fit different car models. This modification minimizes the physical effort required to maneuver in tight spaces and makes entering and exiting a vehicle much more manageable.

- **Sunglasses to reduce eye strain:** Wear quality sunglasses while driving to shield your eyes from glare and reduce eye strain. Choose sunglasses with polarized lenses to minimize reflections and enhance visibility. This small adjustment promotes eye comfort and contributes to safer driving by reducing glare from the sun and other reflective surfaces.

- **Adjustable seat cushions and lumbar support:** Customize your car seat for optimal comfort and support by using adjustable cushions and lumbar support. Experiment with different cushioning options to find the combination that alleviates pressure on your back and enhances your sitting posture. Lumbar support cushions promote a healthy spinal alignment, reducing the risk of discomfort during long drives.

PRO TIP: *For an economical alternative to a lumbar support cushion, roll up a bath towel and place it behind your back where a belt would sit.*

- **Automatic transmission:** If possible, choose a car with an automatic transmission to simplify your driving experience. Automatic vehicles eliminate the need for frequent shifting, reducing the strain on your arms and legs. This modification enhances your driving comfort, especially during stop-and-go traffic or extended periods behind the wheel.
- **Seatbelt adapters:** Ensure that your seatbelt is easy to reach and secure by using a seatbelt adapter. These adapters can extend the length of the seatbelt, making it more accessible and reducing the need for awkward reaching or twisting. They can also make it much simpler to fasten and release the seatbelt, reducing muscle strain in your hands and arms. Invest in seatbelt adapters that are compatible with your car model to enhance safety and ease of use.
- **Organize car essentials for easy access:** Minimize the need to reach and bend while driving by organizing your car essentials strategically. Use a floorboard, center console, or backseat organizer to keep items within arm's reach, preventing the strain (and danger!) of searching for belongings while on the road.

- **Consider hand controls for driving:** Explore the option of hand controls for driving, especially if leg strength or coordination is a concern. Hand controls allow you to operate the accelerator and brake using your hands, providing an alternative and accessible driving solution. Consult with an adaptive driving professional to assess your eligibility and find the best hand control system for your specific needs.
- **Measures to avoid overheating:** Take proactive steps to prevent overheating in your car in hot climates. Use a sunshade to shield your vehicle's interior from direct sunlight, reducing the temperature inside. Additionally, consider installing a remote start system that allows you to initiate the air conditioning before entering the car. This pre-cooling feature minimizes the time you spend in a hot environment, ensuring a more comfortable and temperature-regulated driving experience, especially during warm weather.

By incorporating these life hacks into your car routine, you can create a driving environment that prioritizes comfort, accessibility, and safety. Experiment with different modifications to discover the combination that best suits your needs, making each journey a more enjoyable and accommodating experience.

Household Chore Hacks

- **Use adaptive cleaning tools:** Explore adaptive cleaning tools designed to accommodate individuals with varying levels of strength and coordination. Look for ergonomic broom handles, lightweight vacuum attachments, and specially designed scrub brushes that minimize strain on your hands and arms. Additionally, incorporate long-handled cleaning tools into your arsenal, such as extended mops, dusters, and scrubbers, to reduce the need for bending and reaching. These tools enable you to clean high and low surfaces without exerting unnecessary strain on your muscles.

- **Delegate tasks to others:** Embrace the power of delegation to lighten the load of household chores. Don't hesitate to ask for help from family members or consider hiring a cleaning service for more extensive tasks, if possible. Delegating allows you to distribute responsibilities, ensuring that the physical demands of chores are shared. This collaborative approach not only eases the burden on your body but also promotes a supportive and shared living environment.

- **Implement a chore schedule:** Create a schedule that distributes tasks evenly throughout the week or month. This structured approach prevents the accumulation of chores and allows you to allocate time and energy effectively. A chore schedule also provides a sense of predictability, helping you plan and manage your activities without the stress of last-minute cleaning sessions.

- **Take breaks and pace yourself:** Prioritize your well-being by incorporating breaks and pacing into your chore routine. Avoid the temptation to tackle all tasks at once. Instead, break up your cleaning sessions into smaller, manageable chunks. Set a timer or use task-oriented apps to remind yourself to take breaks at regular intervals. Pacing yourself helps prevent overexertion and allows you to maintain energy levels throughout the cleaning process.

- **Use a laundry basket with wheels:** Carrying a heavy basket can overtax your arms and back, so opt for a basket with built-in wheels for easy maneuverability. This practical solution allows you to roll your laundry from room to room without the physical strain of lifting and carrying. Choose a design with a comfortable handle for a hassle-free and energy-conserving laundry routine.
- **Explore lightweight vacuum options:** Upgrade your vacuum cleaner to a lightweight model that eases the effort required for carpet and floor cleaning. Modern vacuum cleaners come in various designs, some of which are specifically crafted to be lightweight and easy to maneuver. Look for features such as adjustable handles and attachments that cater to different surfaces. A lightweight vacuum makes cleaning more accessible and less physically demanding. Or go one further and invest in a robotic vacuum cleaner!
- **Organize cleaning supplies for easy access:** Arrange your cleaning supplies in an organized manner to reduce the time and effort spent searching for items. Use caddies, baskets, or storage containers to group similar cleaning products together. This simple organization hack ensures that everything you need is easily accessible, minimizing unnecessary movements and making your cleaning routine more efficient.
- **Embrace the "one-in, one-out" rule:** Maintain a clutter-free living space by adopting the "one-in, one-out" rule. For every new item that enters your home, consider removing or donating an existing item. This approach prevents the accumulation of unnecessary belongings, reducing the overall maintenance and cleaning requirements. Embracing simplicity in your

Some Spoons Are Worth Spending

living space contributes to a more manageable and stress-free household environment.

By incorporating these household chore hacks into your routine, you can create an environment that supports both cleanliness and your well-being. Experiment with different strategies to find the combination that best aligns with your needs. This will make household chores more manageable and less energy-expensive, allowing you to maintain a comfortable and organized living space.

❄

Living with MG may present challenges, but with some creativity and practical life hacks, you can make your daily life easier and more comfortable. By implementing these modifications, adaptations, and shortcuts, you can conserve your physical energy, avoid unnecessary strain or stress on your body, and improve your overall quality of life. Remember to listen to your body, take breaks when needed, and don't be afraid to ask for help when necessary. With these strategies in your arsenal, you can save your precious spoons and continue to live a fulfilling and manageable life with MG.

Chapter 5

Exercising Safely

I WOULDN'T BE MUCH OF A PHYSICAL THERAPIST IF I didn't address movement, physical activity, and exercise... And before I go any further, I need to preface this chapter. First, everyone's experience with Myasthenia Gravis (MG) is different, and, specifically, everyone's experience with exercise and physical activity with MG is different, too. The information provided in this chapter is meant to be a ***general guideline only***. For more specific and tailored guidance, please consult your friendly physical therapist. And second, the information in this chapter is in no way exhaustive. (Though some may find it exhausting...) This chapter is one of the longest in the book, but I could honestly write an entirely separate book on this topic alone. So, this chapter is only meant to brush the surface of the topic of MG and exercise.

Now that's out of the way...

❄

UNDERSTANDING MG AND PHYSICAL ACTIVITY

Living with MG presents unique challenges regarding exercise and movement. (Understatement of the century!) Yet, incorporating physical activity into your daily routine can significantly enhance your overall well-being and quality of life. In this chapter, we'll explore the profound impact of physical activity on managing MG symptoms and why it's not merely beneficial but *essential* for individuals navigating this condition.

MG Overview

MG is an autoimmune disorder characterized by muscle weakness and fatigue. The hallmark of MG is the fluctuating nature of symptoms, with periods of weakness followed by periods of relative strength. MG-related muscle weakness is brought on by the immune system's misguided assault on the neuromuscular junction, causing a disruption in the transmission of nerve impulses to muscles.[1]

Think of your muscles like a mobile phone. Your phone is on and charged, and the cellular tower is transmitting. However, you're trying to talk on one bar of signal. Good luck having a conversation!

Impact of MG on Physical Function

MG-related muscle weakness and fatigue present considerable obstacles to mobility, strength, and endurance. Simple tasks that were once relatively easy may now require significant effort and energy. Individuals with MG often encounter challenges in mobility and activities of daily living (ADLs), such as walking, lifting objects,

---

1. U.S. Department of Health and Human Services. (2024). Myasthenia Gravis. National Institute of Neurological Disorders and Stroke. http://www.ninds.nih.gov/health-information/disorders/myasthenia-gravis

climbing stairs, and maintaining balance. Furthermore, the involvement of muscles critical for essential bodily functions, including swallowing and breathing, making everyday activities more complicated.

Importance of Maintaining Physical Activity Despite MG

Despite these challenges, staying physically active is crucial when you have MG. Regular exercise can help improve your muscle strength, endurance, and flexibility, which can make daily tasks easier and help you stay more independent. Exercise also benefits your heart, lifts your mood, and reduces stress—important factors when managing a chronic condition like MG. Additionally, staying active aids in weight management, promotes bone health, and reduces the risk of developing other diseases associated with a sedentary lifestyle.

It's important to approach exercise with caution and adapt activities to fit your abilities. But the rewards of staying active, like better overall health and a more positive outlook, are well worth it. By understanding how MG affects your body and learning safe ways to stay active, you can better manage your condition, maintain your health, and continue to enjoy physical activities that you love.

❄

SAFETY CONSIDERATIONS FOR EXERCISE WITH MG

Safety must be a top priority when integrating exercise into your daily routine. Because of MG's hallmark muscle fatigue that worsens with use and the fluctuating nature of the condition, special care must be taken to ensure that exercise is both safe and effective. "Traditional" exercise guidelines don't always apply to MG and can, in some cases, be dangerous, causing a severe worsening of the condition.

So, first things first...

Consult with Your Healthcare Providers Before Starting an Exercise Program

I'll say it again. **CONSULT WITH YOUR HEALTHCARE PROVIDERS BEFORE STARTING AN EXERCISE PROGRAM.**

Before you start an exercise routine, it's important to talk to your healthcare team. At a minimum, this should include your treating neurologist and a physical therapist. They can help you figure out your current fitness level, understand how MG affects you specifically, and determine if you're ready for physical activity. They can also suggest the best types of exercises for you. This step is crucial to ensure you're safe and get the most benefit from your exercise routine.

- **Importance of Consultation:** Before starting any exercise program, it's essential to consult with your healthcare team, including your neurologist and physical therapist. (Have I said it enough yet?) They can provide valuable insights into your current health status, MG symptoms, and any potential risks associated with exercise.
- **Guidance from Healthcare Professionals:** Your healthcare providers can offer personalized advice on the types of exercises that are safe and beneficial for you, considering the specific nature of your MG symptoms and overall health. They can also recommend appropriate intensity levels and help you set realistic goals for your exercise program.

- **Regular Communication:** Maintain open and ongoing communication with your healthcare team throughout your exercise journey. Provide updates on your progress, any changes in symptoms or medication, and any challenges or concerns you encounter. Your healthcare providers can offer guidance and adjustments to your exercise plan as needed to ensure your safety and well-being.

Identify Appropriate Exercise Types and Intensity Levels

Choosing the right types and intensity levels of exercise is crucial for individuals with MG to reap the benefits of physical activity without worsening symptoms.

- **Recommended Exercises:** Focus on exercises that improve muscle strength, endurance, flexibility, and balance. Low-impact activities such as walking, swimming, tai chi, and gentle or restorative yoga are generally well-tolerated by individuals with MG. Avoid high-impact or strenuous activities that may strain your muscles excessively.
- **Gradual Progression:** Start slowly and gradually increase the intensity and duration of your exercises as your strength and stamina improve. Listen to your body and avoid pushing yourself too hard, especially when your symptoms are worse or you're feeling tired.
- **Listen to Your Body:** Pay close attention to your body's signals during exercise. If you experience excessive muscle weakness, fatigue, difficulty breathing, or other symptoms of MG, stop exercising and rest. It's essential

to honor your body's limits and modify your exercise routine as needed to stay safe and healthy.

Recognize the Warning Signs of Overexertion or Exacerbation of MG Symptoms

Knowing the warning signs of overexertion or worsening MG symptoms is crucial for staying safe during exercise.

- **Common Warning Signs:** Be aware of common warning signs that may indicate overexertion or exacerbation of MG symptoms, such as increased muscle weakness, fatigue, difficulty breathing, changes in speech or swallowing, or a decline in overall function.
- **Action Steps:** If you experience any warning signs during exercise, stop immediately and rest. Take note of your symptoms and consult your healthcare provider if they persist or worsen. Don't push through symptoms or ignore warning signs, as this can lead to more serious problems.
- **Importance of Pacing and Rest:** Pace yourself during exercise and take regular breaks to rest and recover. Include rest periods in your exercise routine to prevent fatigue and minimize the risk of overexertion. Remember that rest is just as important as exercise for staying healthy.

Incorporate Rest Periods into Exercise Routines

Including rest periods in your exercise routines is essential for managing fatigue and preventing overexertion, particularly for individuals with MG.

- **Significance of Rest:** Rest periods allow your muscles to recover, prevent fatigue, and reduce the risk of overexertion. Take short breaks between sets or exercises and longer breaks between workout sessions. Even if you feel fine, don't skip the rest breaks!
- **Structuring Exercise Sessions:** Plan your exercise sessions to include periods of activity and rest. Break up your workout into smaller segments with rest breaks in between. Listen to your body and adjust the duration and intensity of your exercises based on how you feel.
- **Mindfulness and Listening to Your Body:** Listen to your body's signals during exercise. If you feel tired or fatigued, take a break and rest. Avoid pushing yourself too hard or ignoring signs of fatigue, as this can lead to injury or exacerbation of MG symptoms. Respect your body's limits and prioritize your safety and well-being above all else.

❄

OVERCOMING BARRIERS TO EXERCISE

Exercise offers many benefits for people with MG but also comes with unique challenges. Overcoming these barriers requires education, support, and personalized strategies. This section will address common concerns about exercising with MG, ways to seek support, and practical tips for managing symptoms and fatigue during physical activity.

Addressing Common Concerns and Misconceptions about Exercise with MG

Many people with MG feel apprehensive about adding exercise to their routines due to concerns about fatigue and muscle weakness. (Understandably so!) Understanding these concerns is crucial for developing a safe and effective exercise plan.

- **Fear of Worsening Symptoms:** The fear of worsening symptoms or triggering a myasthenic crisis can be daunting. (Again, understandably so!) But with the right guidance and adjustments, you can safely include exercise in your routine. Knowing how tailored exercise can help manage symptoms and improve overall health can ease these fears.

- **Uncertainty About Suitable Activities:** Figuring out which exercises are safe for MG can be challenging. Clearing up misconceptions and getting advice on low-impact, adaptive exercises that match your abilities can help you explore different activities with confidence.

- **Concerns About Fatigue and Energy Levels:** Fatigue is a common MG symptom and can discourage you from being active. However, regular exercise can boost your energy levels and reduce fatigue over time.[2] Start with manageable activities and slowly increase intensity to build stamina and resilience. (Start low and go slow.)

---

2. Veenhuizen, Y., Cup, E. H. C., Jonker, M. A., Voet, N. B. M., van Keulen, B. J., Maas, D. M., Heeren, A., Groothuis, J. T., van Engelen, B. G. M., & Geurts, A. C. H. (2019). Self-management program improves participation in patients with neuromuscular disease: A randomized controlled trial. Neurology, 93(18), e1720–e1731. https://doi.org/10.1212/WNL.0000000000008393

Finding Support from Healthcare Professionals, Support Groups, or Online Communities

Navigating the complexities of exercise with MG often requires support from various sources.

- **Consult with Healthcare Professionals:** Seeking guidance from physicians, physical therapists, or exercise specialists can provide invaluable support and personalized recommendations for safe and effective exercise. They can assess your individual needs, monitor your progress, and address any concerns or challenges that arise.
- **Support Groups:** Connecting with others who understand the challenges of living with MG can offer valuable support, encouragement, and practical advice. Local support groups or online communities dedicated to MG provide a space to share experiences, exchange tips, and find support in your exercise journey.
- **Online Resources:** Accessing reliable online resources, such as online journal articles, educational websites, or *well-moderated* social media groups focused on MG and exercise, can expand knowledge, foster community, and provide inspiration for incorporating physical activity into daily life. Engaging with credible sources and reputable organizations ensures access to accurate information and supportive networks.

Developing Strategies to Overcome Fatigue and Manage Symptoms During Exercise

Exercising with MG can be daunting, but with mindful strategies and a personalized approach, you can safely include physical activity in your routine.

- **Pace and Listen to Your Body:** Pay attention to signs of fatigue or muscle weakness and adjust the intensity or duration of your exercise accordingly. Gradually increase exercise intensity and respect your limits to avoid overexertion and minimize symptom flare-ups.
- **Build in Rest and Recovery:** Include rest breaks in your routine to allow for adequate recovery. Prioritize sleep, hydration, and nutrition to support muscle repair. Balancing activity with rest helps maintain well-being and prevent symptoms from worsening.
- **Implement Symptom Management Strategies:** Use techniques like medication management (with your physician's guidance), stress reduction, and relaxation exercises to manage symptoms during exercise. Consulting healthcare providers for personalized strategies can improve exercise tolerance.
- **Utilize Adaptive Strategies:** Adjust the intensity, duration, or type of exercise to fit your needs. Use assistive devices or adaptive equipment for safety and accessibility.
- **Go at Your Own Pace**: Don't compare your progress to others. Everyone is on their own MG journey. (I can't overstate this!) Recognize and respect your unique limits, celebrating your milestones and improvements. This individualized approach ensures steady, safe progress toward better health and well-being.

By addressing concerns, seeking support, and using tailored strategies, you can overcome barriers to exercise and enjoy a safe, effective, and sustainable physical activity routine. Embracing a holistic approach with education, empowerment, and community support fosters resilience and helps you thrive despite the challenges of MG. Remember, every step toward safe physical activity is a step toward better health and quality of life.

❄

TYPES OF EXERCISES RECOMMENDED FOR MG

Designing a tailored MG-friendly exercise program involves selecting appropriate exercises that enhance muscle strength, endurance, flexibility, and overall physical function while decreasing the risk of worsening symptoms.[3] This section explores various types of exercises recommended for individuals living with MG, their benefits, and practical guidance for implementation.

Low-Impact Aerobic Exercises

Low-impact aerobic exercises offer a gentle yet effective way to improve cardiovascular fitness and overall health without placing excessive stress on the muscles and joints.

- **Walking:** Walking is a highly accessible and adaptable form of exercise for individuals with MG. It can be performed at a comfortable pace, and the intensity can be easily adjusted to suit individual fitness levels. Start with short walks and gradually increase duration and intensity over time.

---

3. Gilhus N. E. (2021). Physical training and exercise in myasthenia gravis. *Neuromuscular disorders : NMD*, 31(3), 169–173. https://doi.org/10.1016/j.nmd.2020.12.004

- **Swimming:** Swimming provides a full-body workout while minimizing impact on the joints. The buoyancy of water reduces the strain on muscles and allows for smooth, controlled movements. Consider incorporating swimming or water-based exercises into your routine to improve cardiovascular endurance and muscle strength.

Resistance Training

Resistance training helps build muscle strength and endurance, which are essential for maintaining functional independence and mobility.

- **Bodyweight Exercises:** Bodyweight exercises are a great place to start because they can be performed without the need for any additional equipment and can be tailored to be as easy or as difficult as you need them to be. These exercises target multiple muscle groups and can be modified to accommodate varying levels of strength and mobility. Easier bodyweight exercises include seated arm raises, seated or standing heel raises, marching, and wall push-ups. Examples of more challenging exercises include squats, lunges, push-ups, and planks.
- **Resistance Bands:** Resistance bands are versatile, portable, and provide variable resistance to challenge the muscles. They can be used to perform a wide range of resistance exercises, including bicep curls, shoulder presses, and leg extensions. Include resistance band exercises in your routine to improve muscle strength and endurance. Resistance bands can be a great progression when bodyweight exercises alone no longer provide enough of a challenge.

- **Light Hand Weights:** Utilize light hand weights or household items such as water bottles or soup cans to add resistance to strength training exercises. Start with low weights and gradually increase as tolerated, focusing on proper form and controlled movements.

Flexibility Exercises

Flexibility exercises help maintain joint mobility, reduce stiffness, and prevent injury, making them essential components of any exercise program.

- **Stretching:** Static and dynamic stretching exercises can help improve flexibility and range of motion. Perform gentle stretches for major muscle groups, focusing on areas prone to tightness. Aim to hold each stretch for 20-30 seconds and repeat 2-3 times.
- **Yoga:** Yoga combines physical postures, breathing exercises, and meditation to promote strength, flexibility, and relaxation. Choose gentle yoga poses that emphasize proper alignment and breath awareness. Modify poses as needed to accommodate any physical limitations or discomfort. (NOTE: People with MG may find sustained yoga poses difficult and potentially fatiguing. Opt for a yoga flow instead, moving between 3-4 different poses to prevent prolonged muscle contraction.)

Balance and Coordination Exercises

Balance and coordination exercises help improve stability,

proprioception, and postural control, reducing the risk of falls and enhancing overall safety.[4]

- **Proprioception Exercises:** Proprioception exercises challenge the body's ability to sense its position in space and make adjustments accordingly. Perform exercises such as standing on one leg, heel-to-toe walking, and balance board exercises to improve proprioceptive awareness and stability. (NOTE: When performing balancing exercises, have something nearby to hold onto for support if needed to avoid falling.)
- **Tai Chi:** Tai Chi is a gentle form of martial arts characterized by slow, flowing movements and deep breathing. It improves balance, coordination, and body awareness while promoting relaxation and stress reduction. Practice Tai Chi movements to enhance balance and coordination in a safe and controlled manner.

PRO TIP: *Tai Chi, among many things, focuses on generating the most movement with the least energy expenditure. Tai Chi is energy conservation in motion, which is why it's so MG-friendly!*

Aquatic Exercises

Aquatic exercises offer a unique opportunity to engage in low-impact workouts while taking advantage of the buoyancy and resistance provided by water. It's also an excellent way to keep cool while exercising and one of my favorite ways to work out.

---

4. Wong, S. H., Nitz, J. C., Williams, K., & Brauer, S. G. (2014). Effects of balance strategy training in myasthenia gravis: a case study series. *Muscle & nerve*, *49*(5), 654–660. https://doi.org/10.1002/mus.24054

- **Precautions:** Before engaging in aquatic exercises, consult with your healthcare provider to ensure they are safe for your individual condition. Start in shallow water where you can touch the bottom, and gradually progress to deeper water as your confidence and ability improve. Use a flotation belt or device to maintain buoyancy and support during aquatic activities. Be sure to take it easy, as the buoyancy of the water can mask muscle fatigue, so your muscles may be more fatigued than you think. For the same reason, take special care when exiting the pool, as you may be more tired than you thought.
- **Water-Based Exercises:** Try water-based exercises such as water walking, leg lifts, arm circles, and water aerobics to improve cardiovascular fitness, muscle strength, and flexibility. The resistance provided by water adds an extra challenge to your workouts while reducing stress on your joints.
- **Swimming:** Gentle lap swimming or treading water is a great way to get a low-impact, full-body workout that builds muscle strength and endurance, cardiorespiratory endurance, and joint mobility in one exercise. The buoyancy of the water supports the body, reducing the risk of injury and muscle fatigue while allowing for a wider range of motion. Additionally, the rhythmic breathing required in swimming can improve respiratory function, which is particularly beneficial for those with MG. When starting, opt for a more energy-efficient stroke like breaststroke. Alternate strokes to target different muscle groups. Be sure to rest between laps to prevent fatigue.

Incorporating a variety of exercises into your routine can help you reap the benefits of physical activity while managing the symptoms of MG. Remember to listen to your body, pace yourself, and consult with your healthcare provider before starting any new exercise program. With careful planning and proper guidance, you can enjoy the many benefits of exercise while effectively managing your MG symptoms.

❄

STRATEGIES FOR EXERCISING SAFELY WITH MG

Exercising safely with MG requires some careful planning to manage the unique challenges of the condition. In this section, we will explore strategies to help you enjoy the benefits of physical activity while minimizing the risk of worsening your symptoms.

Warm-up and Cool-down Routines

- **Importance of Warm-up:** Starting your exercise routine with a proper warm-up is good advice in general but especially important for individuals with MG. The warm-up phase gradually elevates your heart rate, increases blood flow to the muscles, and enhances joint flexibility, reducing the risk of injury and improving performance. Try dynamic stretches, gentle cardio activities, and mobility exercises to prepare your body for the upcoming workout.
- **Cool-down Techniques:** Just as warming up is crucial, cooling down post-exercise is equally essential for a safe and effective workout. Cooling down aids in gradually reducing heart rate and blood pressure and helps remove metabolic waste products from the muscles. Incorporate

static stretches targeting major muscle groups, gentle movements, and deep breathing exercises to promote relaxation and aid in recovery.

Use Assistive Devices or Adaptive Equipment as Needed

- **Assistive Devices:** If you have mobility issues or balance problems, using assistive devices can provide support during exercise. Walkers, canes, or stability poles can give you better balance and stability, reducing the risk of falls. Talk to your healthcare provider (ideally, a physical therapist) to find the right device for your needs and preferences.
- **Adaptive Equipment:** Adaptations and modifications to exercise equipment can make exercise safer and more accessible. Consider using resistance bands instead of traditional weights to control resistance levels and minimize the risk of muscle strain. Ergonomic equipment, such as adjustable benches or supportive cushions, can improve comfort and stability during strength training exercises.

Modify Exercises to Accommodate Fluctuating Energy Levels

- **Avoid Repetitive or Sustained Contractions:** Long or repetitive muscle contractions can quickly lead to fatigue and worsen MG symptoms. Mix up your exercises to target different muscle groups and movement patterns. Circuit-style workouts or alternating between resistance training and cardio exercises can give you adequate rest intervals and prevent overexertion.

- **Rotate Muscle Groups:** Switching between different muscle groups during your workout can help maintain endurance and reduce fatigue. Alternate between upper body, lower body, and core exercises to distribute the workload evenly and avoid overworking specific muscle groups.
- **Consider Circuits:** Circuit training allows you to move smoothly between different exercises, giving muscle groups relative rest. Design your circuit workouts to include a mix of strength, cardio, and flexibility exercises. This method ensures you get a full-body workout with adequate recovery time between sets.

Monitor Symptoms and Adjust Exercise Intensity Accordingly

- **Time Exercise for Higher Energy Levels:** Identify times of the day when your energy levels are typically higher and schedule your workouts accordingly. Whether it's morning, afternoon, or evening, pick a time when you feel most energetic and ready to exercise.
- **Take Frequent Rest Breaks:** Include rest breaks in your exercise routine to manage fatigue and prevent symptom flare-ups. Listen to your body and take short, frequent breaks to rest and recover. Don't wait until you feel exhausted; take preemptive breaks to keep your energy levels up.
- **Rest Before You Think You Need To:** Resting before you reach the point of exhaustion is crucial with MG. Since symptoms can come on suddenly, it's best to rest

proactively. Listen to your body and take breaks to avoid overexertion and conserve energy.

Exercise in a Cool and Dry Environment to Avoid Overheating

- **Cool and Dry Environment:** Exercising in a cool, well-ventilated place helps prevent overheating and reduces the risk of worsening your MG symptoms. Choose indoor facilities with air conditioning or well-shaded outdoor areas for your workouts.
- **Stay Hydrated:** Keeping hydrated is vital for maintaining exercise performance and regulating body temperature. Drink water before, during, and after exercise to replace fluids lost through sweat. Watch for signs of dehydration, like dry mouth, dizziness, or dark urine, and make sure you drink enough to stay hydrated.

By using these strategies, you can safely and effectively navigate the challenges of exercising with MG. Always prioritize your safety, listen to your body, and consult with a healthcare professional to tailor your exercise routine to your needs. With careful planning and adaptation, you can enjoy the many benefits of exercise and improve your overall health and well-being despite the challenges of MG.

❄

CASE STUDIES: REAL-LIFE EXAMPLES OF EXERCISE SUCCESS STORIES WITH MG

It's one thing to read about the clinical and textbook benefits of exercise but quite another to hear real stories about how it's actually helped people living with MG. Through detailed accounts of individuals who were clients of mine, you can see the real challenges they faced, the strategies they employed, and the remarkable outcomes they achieved. (Both clients have given me permission to share their experiences, and I have changed their names to protect their identities.)

Personal Stories Highlighting the Benefits of Exercise for MG Management

Sarah's Journey to Strength

Sarah, a client of mine diagnosed with MG in her early twenties, initially struggled with profound muscle weakness and fatigue. Sarah had been an avid runner through high school and college, and she had a tough time coming to grips with the physical limitations that came with MG. Determined to regain her strength and mobility, Sarah embarked on a comprehensive exercise program tailored to her needs. Under my guidance, she gradually progressed from gentle stretching and mobility exercises to more challenging resistance training and cardiovascular workouts.

Despite facing setbacks and periods of symptom exacerbation, Sarah remained steadfast in her commitment to her exercise regimen. Over time, she began to notice significant improvements in her muscle strength, endurance, and overall energy levels. Today, Sarah leads an active lifestyle, participating in yoga classes, swimming sessions, and regular hikes in nature. While she has not returned to running and may never, she is happy with her "new normal" and can still reap the physical and mental benefits of being physically active. Through her dedication to exercise and wellness, she has not only managed her MG symptoms effectively but also experienced a profound sense of empowerment and vitality.

John's Triumph Over Adversity

John, another client of mine, was diagnosed with MG later in life and initially struggled to come to terms with the challenges posed by the condition. Despite facing numerous setbacks and fluctuations in symptoms, John was determined to reclaim control over his health and well-being. With my guidance and support, he embarked on a tailored exercise program focused on improving muscle strength, balance, and coordination. Through perseverance and resilience, John overcame adversity and achieved remarkable progress in his fitness journey. He discovered a newfound sense of purpose and confidence as he tackled each workout with determination and grit. Over time, John's muscle strength and endurance improved significantly, enabling him to engage in activities he once thought impossible.

Today, John leads an active lifestyle, participating in regular walks, strength training sessions, and swimming laps in his backyard pool. His personal goal was to take his wife out dancing, and I'm happy to report that he was successful. He went from frequently stumbling and barely able to walk to the mailbox to taking his wife country and western dancing on Thursday nights. His journey serves as a testament to the transformative power of exercise in managing MG and embracing life to the fullest.

Challenges and Strategies to Overcome Them

- **Managing Fatigue and Fluctuating Symptoms**: Both Sarah and John encountered challenges related to fatigue and fluctuating symptoms throughout their exercise journey. To overcome these obstacles, they implemented strategies such as pacing themselves, listening to their bodies, and incorporating rest breaks into their exercise routines. By prioritizing self-care and flexibility, they navigated through periods of heightened symptoms while maintaining their commitment to physical activity.

- **Adapting Exercise Routines**: Another challenge for individuals with MG is adapting exercise routines to accommodate their unique needs and capabilities. Sarah and John experimented with various types of exercise, modifying intensity, duration, and frequency as needed. They also utilized assistive devices and adaptive equipment to enhance safety and accessibility during workouts. By embracing adaptability and creativity, they found ways to engage in physical activity that suited their individual preferences and abilities.

My Physical Activity Journey

In addition to guiding clients through their exercise journeys, I also draw from my personal experience with MG to inform and inspire others. As someone living with MG myself, I understand the daily challenges and limitations associated with the condition. However, I refuse to let MG define or restrict me. By prioritizing physical activity and wellness, I have experienced firsthand the profound benefits of exercise in managing symptoms and enhancing quality of life.

One of the most rewarding aspects of being more physically active is the ability to fully engage in activities with my dogs and keep up with the energetic pace of my children. Whether playing fetch in the backyard or walking around the lake with my kids, being active allows me to embrace life's moments with vitality and joy.

I fully accept that I may never have the fitness level I had prior to MG, and I'm okay with that. Before MG, I served in the military—specifically the US Navy. While I admittedly never cared for the running, I did enjoy the military's culture of fitness. I regularly took part in group exercise sessions with my colleagues, including high-intensity interval training and weight lifting. In my youth, I was a competitive swimmer, and I played organized sports (though not very well). Now that I have MG, exercise looks different for me. However, through careful training and dedication, I can still safely enjoy physical activity. Now, physical activity looks more like walks, bike rides, swimming, and moderate-intensity circuit training, but I am still able to reap the health benefits of staying physically active. I hope that by leading by example, my personal journey serves as a testament to the transformative power of exercise in overcoming the obstacles posed by MG and living life to the fullest.

❄

TAKE-HOME POINTS

1. **Start Slow**: Begin with the easiest exercises and gradually progress to more strenuous ones based on comfort and endurance.
2. **Rest Frequently**: Take breaks as needed to avoid overexertion. Rest before you think you need to.
3. **Stay Hydrated**: Keep hydrated to help muscle function and overall health.
4. **Monitor Symptoms**: Pay attention to any signs of fatigue or muscle weakness and adjust exercises accordingly.
5. **Consult a Healthcare Provider**: Always check with a healthcare professional before starting a new exercise regimen to ensure it's safe and appropriate.

Chapter 6

Working

PROFESSIONAL LIFE IS A TOPIC THAT IS NEAR AND DEAR TO my heart. I was raised by two very hard-working entrepreneurial parents, and they instilled in me not only an exceptionally high work ethic but also a passion, joy, and pride in what I choose to devote my life to. For better or worse, my professional life is an essential part of my identity.

When I was diagnosed with Myasthenia Gravis (MG), this was one of the biggest hits to my identity. At the time, I was an active-duty physical therapist in the US Navy. I had a shipboard deployment under my belt, along with a few special duty assignments, and I was in a rigorous leadership role at a medium-sized military medical facility. My plan at the time was to have a full and robust military career, rank up a few more times, and perhaps have a shot at a commanding officer's chair. Then MG happened...

Long story short, MG and a military career are rarely compatible. (I am aware of a few servicemembers who have been able to stay on active duty after being diagnosed with MG, but such was not the case with me.) I went through a painstakingly long physical evaluation board (PEB) that ultimately medically retired me from service. So, I lost my military career.

But it was more than that. My career as a physical therapist was also in jeopardy. Prior to the onset of MG, I was a staunch orthopedic PT with a passion for manual therapy (manually mobilizing joints, muscles, and other soft tissue), which is a physically demanding PT subspeciality. I had worked long and hard for a career that I loved, and the prospect of having to give it up was frankly depressing.

I had to make hard and fast decisions about what working life was going to look like for me. Serendipitously, I came across a podcast about telehealth physical therapy (well before the COVID-19 pandemic popularized telemedicine). After lots of research, collaboration, and trials with willing family and friends, I moved into the telehealth sphere. This was a perfect move for me because it allowed me to continue to see patients but in such a way that respected the limitations of MG. But it also allowed me to reach an underserved patient population—people with chronic pain and fatiguing conditions (like MG!) who needed a better way to access physical therapy than physically going to a brick-and-mortar clinic.

Eventually, I zeroed in on only working with the MG community. So, in a way, my forced change in career path has allowed me to serve a community that needs more dedicated quality care providers. And people say the universe doesn't have a sense of humor...

❄

HOW MG AFFECTS WORKING LIFE

Living with MG can significantly impact one's ability to perform effectively in the workplace. It's essential to understand how MG symptoms can affect work performance and productivity.

Before I get too far into this, however, I would like to highlight that every person's situation is different. People have different jobs, different family and financial situations, and different presentations of MG. I will do my best to be as wide-reaching as possible, but please keep in mind that suggestions for working life are suggestions and examples only and may not apply to your specific situation. Everyone's situation is unique, and it's essential to consider factors such as your disease presentation, financial situation, family and community support, and personal preferences when making decisions about your career path with MG.

Okay, now that's out of the way, let's address the impact of MG symptoms on your ability to work. Fatigable muscle weakness is the most prevalent symptom of MG and a significant challenge faced by individuals with MG in the workplace. Tasks that require physical strength or endurance, such as lifting, carrying, or prolonged standing, can become incredibly difficult or even impossible. Simple actions like typing on a keyboard or holding a pen may also become arduous due to muscle weakness in the hands and arms.

Global fatigue is another MG challenge, often exacerbated by the body's constant struggle with muscle weakness. This fatigue isn't always purely physical; it can also manifest as cognitive fog, making it challenging to concentrate and focus on tasks.

Moreover, the unpredictable nature of MG symptoms means that planning ahead can be difficult. You may experience periods of relative wellness followed by sudden flare-ups, further complicating your ability to maintain consistent productivity. Sudden symptom flare-ups, which can happen despite one's best efforts, may require deferring work commitments or taking unplanned sick leave. This unpredictability can create added stress and anxiety, which doesn't do any favors for MG.

Understanding how MG symptoms can impact your work is the first step toward effectively managing your career while living with this condition. By acknowledging the challenges you face and seeking support and accommodations where necessary, you can take proactive steps to mitigate the impact of MG on your work performance and productivity. Remember, you are not alone in this journey. Resources and support are available to help you navigate the challenges of working with MG.

❄️

ENERGY CONSERVATION STRATEGIES FOR THE WORKPLACE

Managing MG in the workplace requires strategic energy conservation strategies to navigate daily tasks effectively. From prioritizing tasks to leveraging assistive technology, individuals with MG can optimize their work environment to minimize fatigue and maximize productivity. This section explores practical tips and techniques for conserving energy in the workplace and thriving professionally while managing MG's challenges.

Prioritize Tasks

Focus on completing high-priority tasks during periods of peak energy. For some, this might be first thing in the morning, and for others, the early afternoon may be a more energetic time of day. Identify key objectives for the day and allocate your energy resources accordingly to tackle essential tasks when you are feeling at your best. Also, be sure to break down large projects into smaller, manageable tasks to prevent feeling overwhelmed. Use tools like to-do lists or project management software to organize tasks and track your progress.

Manage Your Time

Implement time management techniques such as the Pomodoro Technique[1] or time-blocking to structure your workday into focused intervals with built-in rest breaks. The Pomodoro Technique (a personal favorite of mine) involves working in short, focused bursts (typically 20-25 minutes) followed by a short break. After four Pomodoros, take a longer break. (Note: This technique is named for the Pomodoro [tomato] shaped kitchen timer. Use one to time your work and rest intervals.) Time-blocking involves scheduling specific blocks of time for different tasks or activities throughout the day, allowing you to allocate your energy resources efficiently. These strategies will enable you to maintain productivity while conserving energy and avoiding burnout.

Delegate Responsibilities

Delegate tasks that are not essential to your role or require significant physical or cognitive effort to colleagues or support staff. Distributing workload can lighten your burden and conserve energy for tasks that require your skills and attention.

Use Assistive Technology

Use assistive technology tools and software to streamline tasks, automate processes, and reduce manual effort. Voice-to-text software, speech recognition programs, and keyboard shortcuts can minimize physical strain and fatigue and save time. Consider using automated task management apps or digital calendars to organize and prioritize tasks efficiently.

---

1. Cirillo, F. (2023). The Pomodoro Technique. https://www.pomodorotechnique.com/

Optimize Workspace Ergonomics

Arrange your workspace to promote comfort, efficiency, and ergonomic support. Adjust the height of your chair and desk to maintain proper posture and alignment and reduce strain on your muscles and joints. Position your computer monitor at eye level to reduce neck strain and minimize glare. Use ergonomic accessories such as back support cushions, wrist rests, footrests, and keyboards to enhance comfort and productivity.

> **PRO TIP**: *When seated at the computer, place a firm pillow on your lap to rest your elbows. This can help reduce the work your shoulders must do to raise your arms to reach the keyboard.*

Take Regular Breaks

Incorporate short breaks into your workday to rest and recharge. Step away from your desk, stretch your muscles, and practice mindful breathing exercises or brief meditation sessions to combat physical and mental fatigue. Breaks help prevent overexertion and maintain focus throughout the day. But you have to take them! Set reminders or timers to ensure that you take those regular breaks.

Reduce Eye Strain

Eye muscles tend to fatigue quickly with MG, causing blurry or double vision. This can be incredibly taxing if your job requires lots of computer work. Adjust the brightness, contrast, and font size on your computer monitor to enhance readability and reduce strain on your eyes. Increasing font size and using high-contrast color schemes can make text easier to read. Ensure your workspace is well-lit with natural or adjustable lighting to minimize glare and reduce eye strain.

Position your monitor away from direct light sources to prevent glare, and use window blinds or curtains to control brightness.

> **PRO TIP**: *Follow the 20-20-20 rule to take regular breaks from screen time. Every 20 minutes, look away from your screen and focus on an object at least 20 feet (6 meters) away for 20 seconds. This will help relax your eye muscles and prevent fatigue.*

Communicate Openly

Advocate for your needs and communicate openly with your supervisor or HR department about accommodations that can support your energy conservation efforts. Provide specific examples of how certain accommodations or adjustments can enhance your productivity and well-being. Collaborate with your employer to develop a plan that addresses your needs while meeting the requirements of your role and the organization. Discuss flexible work arrangements, remote work options, or adjustments to your workload to ensure a supportive and accommodating work environment. (See "Workplace Accommodations" below for more information.)

Establish Boundaries

Easier said than done, I know. Set boundaries around your time, energy, and availability to prevent overcommitment and burnout. Learn to prioritize tasks and say "no" to non-essential commitments or requests that may drain your energy reserves unnecessarily. Advocate for yourself assertively but respectfully to ensure colleagues and supervisors respect your boundaries. Only you can prioritize your health and well-being.

Dr. Liz Plowman

Monitor and Adjust

Track your energy levels, productivity, and symptoms over time to identify patterns and adjust your work routine as needed. Experiment with different strategies and techniques to find what works best for you and optimize your energy conservation efforts in the workplace.

❄

WORKPLACE ACCOMMODATIONS

Workplace accommodations can significantly improve your ability to perform your job effectively while managing your MG symptoms. Under the Americans with Disabilities Act (ADA)[2] and similar laws in other countries, employers must provide reasonable accommodations to employees with disabilities, including those with MG. These accommodations are intended to level the playing field and ensure that individuals with disabilities have equal opportunities in the workplace.

Here are some examples of workplace accommodations that you may consider requesting:

- **Flexible Work Schedule**: Ask your employer for flexibility in your work hours to accommodate fluctuations in your energy levels. This could involve adjusting your start and end times, working part-time, or implementing a compressed workweek schedule.
- **Telecommuting Options**: Request the ability to work remotely, either full-time or on specific days of the week.

---

2. US Department of Justice and Civil Rights Division. (2024). The Americans with Disabilities Act (ADA). https://www.ada.gov/

Working from home can reduce the physical and mental strain associated with commuting and provide a more comfortable environment for managing your symptoms.

- **Ergonomic Workspace**: Advocate for ergonomic adjustments to your workspace to minimize physical strain and discomfort. This may include ergonomic chairs, adjustable desks, keyboard trays, and monitor stands to promote proper posture and reduce muscle fatigue.
- **Assistive Technology**: Explore using assistive technology to enhance your productivity and accessibility in the workplace. This could involve screen reader software for individuals with vision impairment, voice-to-text software for those with dexterity limitations, or speech recognition software for hands-free computer operation.
- **Breaks and Rest Periods**: Request regular breaks throughout the day to rest and recharge your energy levels. This could involve short rest breaks between tasks, longer rest periods during peak fatigue times, or the ability to take unscheduled breaks as needed.
- **Job Restructuring**: Work with your employer to restructure your job duties and responsibilities to better align with your abilities and energy levels. This could involve delegating specific tasks to colleagues, redistributing workload priorities, or modifying job tasks to reduce physical or cognitive demands.
- **Environmental Modifications**: Request modifications to your work environment to accommodate your specific needs. This could include no outdoor activities during warmer hours, adjusting lighting levels to reduce glare and eye strain, providing noise-canceling headphones to

minimize distractions, or creating a quiet space for rest breaks.

- **Communication Support**: Ask for accommodations to support effective communication in the workplace. This could involve written communication alternatives for individuals with speech difficulties, preferential seating arrangements for better visibility during meetings, or access to voice recognition software to make typed communication (e.g., emails) easier.

- **Flexible Leave Policies**: Inquire about flexible leave policies that allow for time off as needed to manage your MG symptoms. This could include sick leave, disability leave, or the ability to use accrued paid time off for medical appointments and treatments. In the United States, the Family Medical Leave Act (FMLA)[3] allows up to twelve weeks of protected time off for medical reasons, and other countries have similar protections in place. (See "A Note about FMLA.")

When requesting workplace accommodations, it's essential to communicate openly and collaboratively with your employer. Provide documentation from your healthcare provider outlining your specific limitations and recommended accommodations. Emphasize the benefits of these accommodations in enabling you to perform your job effectively and contribute to the organization's success. By advocating for your needs and working together with your employer, you can create a supportive work environment that enables you to thrive despite the challenges of living with MG.

---

3. US Department of Labor. (2024). Family and medical leave act. US Department of Labor. https://www.dol.gov/agencies/whd/fmla

A Note About FMLA

The Family and Medical Leave Act (FMLA) is a federal law in the United States that provides eligible employees up to 12 weeks of unpaid, job-protected leave per year for specified family and medical reasons. FMLA can be incredibly beneficial for individuals living with MG as it offers protection and flexibility during times when managing the condition requires significant time away from work.

Here's how FMLA can help someone with MG:

- **Medical Leave**: Individuals with MG may experience flare-ups or exacerbations of symptoms that require medical treatment or hospitalization. FMLA allows eligible employees to take unpaid leave for their own serious health condition, including time off for medical appointments, diagnostic testing, treatments such as intravenous immunoglobulin (IVIG) therapy or plasma exchange, and recovery from procedures or surgeries related to MG.
- **Family Care**: In addition to medical leave for their own health needs, individuals with MG may also need to take FMLA leave to care for a family member with a serious health condition. This could include providing support and assistance to a spouse, child, or parent who also has MG or another qualifying medical condition.
- **Intermittent Leave**: FMLA allows eligible employees to take intermittent leave, meaning they can take time off in separate blocks of time or on a reduced schedule when medically necessary. This flexibility is especially valuable for individuals with MG, as symptoms can fluctuate unpredictably, requiring periodic rest or medical treatment.

Dr. Liz Plowman

- **Job Protection**: One of the key benefits of FMLA is job protection. Eligible employees who take FMLA leave are entitled to return to their same position or an equivalent position with equivalent pay, benefits, and other terms and conditions of employment upon their return to work. This provides peace of mind and ensures that individuals with MG do not face retaliation or discrimination for taking necessary time off to manage their health.
- **Documentation**: FMLA requires certification from a healthcare provider to verify the need for medical leave due to a serious health condition. This documentation helps ensure that employees receive the support and accommodations they need to manage their MG effectively and facilitates communication between employees, employers, and healthcare providers.

Overall, FMLA provides essential protections and support for individuals living with MG, allowing them to prioritize their health and well-being without jeopardizing their employment. By taking advantage of FMLA leave when needed, individuals with MG can better manage their symptoms, seek necessary medical care, and maintain a healthy work-life balance.

❄

MODIFYING YOUR PROFESSION

People living with MG are frequently required to adjust their professional lives to accommodate the changes and limitations associated with the condition. Whether you're experiencing muscle weakness, fatigue, or cognitive fog, there are various strategies you can employ to continue working effectively while managing MG symptoms.

Modifying Your Current Job/Profession

- **Assess Your Job Duties**: Evaluate your current job responsibilities and identify tasks that may be challenging due to MG symptoms. Consider whether specific tasks can be delegated to colleagues or modified to reduce physical or cognitive demands.
- **Request Accommodations**: Advocate for workplace accommodations that address your needs, such as ergonomic equipment, flexible work hours, or modified job duties. Communicate openly with your employer about your needs and how accommodations can support your continued productivity and success in your role.
- **Pace Yourself**: Prioritize tasks and allocate your energy wisely throughout the day. Take regular breaks to rest and recharge, and be mindful of your limitations to avoid overexertion.

Decreasing to Part-Time Work

- **Consider Reduced Hours**: If managing a full-time work schedule becomes overwhelming, explore options for reducing your hours to part-time. This allows you to maintain employment while providing more flexibility to manage MG symptoms and prioritize self-care.
- **Negotiate with Your Employer**: Initiate a conversation with your employer about transitioning to a part-time work schedule. Highlight the benefits of this

arrangement, such as improved work-life balance and enhanced productivity during scheduled work hours.

- **Plan Financially**: Assess the financial implications of reducing your work hours and adjust your budget accordingly. Consider factors such as changes in income, benefits eligibility, and any potential impact on retirement savings or insurance coverage.

Working from Home

- **Explore Remote Work Opportunities**: Investigate whether your current employer offers remote work options or consider seeking employment with companies that support telecommuting. Remote work provides flexibility and eliminates the stress of commuting, making it easier to manage MG symptoms from the comfort of home.
- **Set Up a Functional Workspace**: Designate a dedicated workspace in your home that is conducive to productivity and free from distractions. Invest in ergonomic furniture and equipment to support proper posture and minimize physical strain.
- **Establish Boundaries**: Establish clear boundaries between work and personal life to maintain a healthy balance. Set specific work hours, communicate availability to colleagues, and resist the temptation to work outside of designated hours to prevent burnout. (As an avid work-from-home enthusiast, I can't emphasize this enough!)

Stopping Work Altogether

- **Assess Your Health Needs**: If MG symptoms significantly impact your ability to work, consider whether taking a temporary or permanent leave of absence is necessary. Consult with your healthcare provider to evaluate your health status and determine the best course of action.
- **Explore Disability Benefits**: Investigate options for disability benefits, such as Social Security Disability Insurance (SSDI)[4] in the United States or its equivalent in your country. Depending on your benefits package, you may have access to long-term disability insurance through your employer. Determine your eligibility criteria and the application process to ensure financial support during periods of unemployment.
- **Focus on Self-Care**: Prioritize self-care and focus on managing MG symptoms effectively during periods of unemployment. Develop a routine that includes regular movement and activity, healthy eating, adequate rest, and social support to maintain overall well-being.

Ultimately, modifying your profession with MG requires careful consideration of your individual needs, preferences, and limitations. By proactively exploring accommodation options, adjusting work arrangements, and prioritizing self-care, you can navigate the challenges of MG while continuing to pursue meaningful employment and career fulfillment.

❄

---

4. Social Security Administration. (2024). Disability. Social Security. https://www.ssa.gov/disability

EXPLORING NEW CAREER FIELDS

If modifying your current profession simply isn't an option, consider transitioning to a new career field that better accommodates your needs and limitations. While changing career paths can be a significant decision, it can also open up opportunities for personal and professional growth while managing MG symptoms effectively. Here are some considerations for exploring new career fields with MG:

- **Assess Your Skills and Interests**: Reflect on your skills, strengths, and interests to identify potential career paths that align with your abilities and passions. Consider your past experiences, educational background, and transferable skills that can be applied to new roles or industries. Research various career fields and industries to gain insights into job opportunities, requirements, and growth prospects. Look for roles that offer flexibility, remote work options, or accommodations that can support your MG management needs.
- **Seek Vocational Guidance and Support**: Seek guidance from vocational rehabilitation counselors or career coaches who specialize in assisting individuals with disabilities. They can provide valuable insights, resources, and support to help you navigate the career exploration process and identify suitable job opportunities. Take advantage of job placement services offered by disability advocacy organizations, vocational training programs, or government agencies. These services can connect you with employers who are committed to diversity, inclusion, and accommodating individuals with disabilities.

- **Consider Remote Work Opportunities**: Remote work offers flexibility and accessibility for individuals with MG who may need to manage symptoms from home. Look for remote job opportunities in fields such as customer service, administration, writing, or virtual assistance that can be performed remotely with minimal physical exertion. Utilize online job boards, freelance marketplaces, and networking platforms to search for remote work opportunities and connect with employers who offer telecommuting options. Tailor your résumé and cover letter to highlight your remote work experience and skills relevant to the position.

- **Pursue Educational and Training Opportunities (Upskill or Re-skill)**: Consider enrolling in educational programs, workshops, or online courses to enhance your skills and qualifications in your desired career field. Look for classes that offer flexible scheduling, self-paced learning, or accommodations for individuals with disabilities. Investigate vocational training programs or apprenticeships that provide hands-on experience and practical skills training in industries such as healthcare, technology, or skilled trades. These programs offer opportunities to gain valuable experience and transition into new career fields.

- **Network and Build Professional Relationships**: Join professional associations or networking groups related to your target career field. Attend industry events, webinars, and networking opportunities to connect with professionals, learn about job openings, and gain insights into industry trends. Seek out mentors or advisors who can provide guidance, support, and advice as you navigate your career transition. Reach out to individuals who have successfully transitioned into your desired career field or who have experience working with individuals with disabilities.

Transitioning to a new career field with MG may present challenges, but it also offers personal and professional growth opportunities. By assessing your skills, exploring new career options, seeking support from vocational resources, and leveraging remote work opportunities, you can embark on a fulfilling career path that aligns with your abilities and accommodates your MG management needs.

❄

SELF-EMPLOYMENT

Self-employment can offer several benefits for individuals living with MG, providing greater flexibility, autonomy, and control over work arrangements and accommodations. I realize not everyone has the entrepreneurial spark. (I've had it since I was eight and discovered the neighbors would pay me to wash their cars.) Honestly, being self-employed has turned out to be the best situation personally for managing my MG. So, if you're like me and have the drive to be self-employed, here are some ways self-employment may benefit someone with MG:

- **Flexible Work Schedule**: Self-employment allows individuals to create their own work schedules, making it easier to accommodate fluctuations in energy levels and manage MG symptoms. They can schedule work tasks during times of the day when they feel most alert and productive and take breaks as needed to rest and recharge.

- **Customized Work Environment**: Self-employed individuals have the freedom to design their work environment to suit their needs and preferences. They can set up a home office with ergonomic furniture and equipment, adjust lighting levels to reduce glare and eye strain, and create a quiet and comfortable workspace conducive to productivity and well-being.
- **Reduced Commuting Stress**: Working from home as a self-employed individual eliminates the need for daily commutes to and from an office, reducing stress and physical exertion associated with transportation. This can be especially beneficial for individuals with MG who may experience fatigue or muscle weakness that makes commuting challenging.
- **Accommodation Flexibility**: If you are self-employed, you are your own boss! Therefore, you can implement accommodations and modifications tailored to your specific needs and limitations due to MG. You can adjust work tasks, schedule rest breaks, and change your workflow to manage symptoms effectively and maintain productivity.
- **Diverse Income Streams**: Self-employment offers the opportunity to diversify income streams and explore multiple sources of revenue. Individuals with MG can pursue various freelance gigs, consulting projects, or entrepreneurial ventures that align with their skills and interests, providing financial stability and independence.
- **Control Over Workload**: Self-employed individuals have the autonomy to control their workload and pace themselves according to their energy levels and health status. They can take on projects at their own discretion, negotiate deadlines and deliverables, and prioritize tasks based on their capacity to handle them effectively.

- **Entrepreneurial Opportunities**: Self-employment opens up entrepreneurial opportunities for individuals with MG to start their own businesses or ventures. They can pursue ventures that cater to their interests and passions while leveraging their skills and expertise to create value for others. This could include launching an online store, offering consulting services, or providing specialized services tailored to their niche market.

Overall, self-employment can provide individuals with MG greater flexibility, independence, and control over their work arrangements. This allows them to effectively manage their symptoms while pursuing meaningful and fulfilling work opportunities. By embracing self-employment, individuals with MG can create a work-life balance that promotes health, well-being, and professional success.

❄

Mastering energy conservation strategies in the workplace is vital for individuals living and working with MG. By implementing practical tips such as prioritizing tasks, utilizing assistive technology, and setting boundaries, you can optimize your work environment to minimize fatigue and maximize productivity. It's essential to recognize that everyone's journey with MG is unique, and choosing the work situation that works best for you is crucial. Whether it involves modifying a current job, changing careers, dropping to part-time, working from home, working for yourself, or retiring altogether, prioritizing self-care and advocating for your needs is paramount.

Remember, managing MG in the workplace requires patience, flexibility, and a willingness to explore different options. With dedication and perseverance, you can create a fulfilling and sustainable work-life balance that supports your health and well-being.

Chapter 7

Traveling

TRAVELING HAS ALWAYS BEEN A PASSION OF MINE. I WAS always the kid excited to get on an airplane. Truth be told, I'm still that kid! (A significant portion of this book was actually written on an airplane or in an airport lounge.) Living with MG has meant making some travel adjustments to accommodate my condition. In this chapter, I'll share tips and strategies for navigating travel with MG. While it can be challenging, I've found that the rewards of exploring new places and cultures far outweigh the obstacles.

Whether you're traveling for personal enrichment or professional growth, each journey is a testament to the resilience and spirit of those of us with MG. Exploring new cultures and environments can be deeply rewarding, enhancing your well-being and opening doors to new opportunities. By approaching travel with a bit of planning and flexibility, you can create memorable experiences that transcend the limitations of MG. This chapter is here to help you make the most of your travels, ensuring your adventures are as enjoyable and enriching as possible.

❄

BEFORE YOU GO: UNDERSTANDING YOUR NEEDS AND RESEARCHING YOUR HEALTHCARE OPTIONS

Embarking on a journey with MG requires a comprehensive understanding of personal challenges and a proactive approach to address specific needs during travel. Before venturing into new destinations, it is crucial to reflect on your unique requirements and consult healthcare professionals to ensure a well-prepared and enjoyable trip.

Reflect on Personal MG Challenges

Begin by assessing the specific challenges MG poses in your daily life. Reflect on your energy levels, potential triggers, and any recent changes in symptoms. Understanding how MG manifests in your individual case will inform the strategies needed to navigate travel successfully.

Consult with Healthcare Professionals

Reach out to your healthcare team well in advance of your trip. Discuss your travel plans, and seek guidance on managing MG symptoms during the journey. Your healthcare provider can provide valuable insights, adjust medications if necessary, and offer recommendations to enhance your overall well-being while away from home.

Research Healthcare Options at Your Destination

Investigate healthcare options at your destination, ensuring you are aware of available medical facilities and services. Research local hospitals, clinics, and MG specialists in the area. Additionally, explore the availability of assistive devices or mobility aids that may be required during your stay.

Insurance Coverage

Check the terms of your health insurance policy to see if you are covered for medical care while traveling. Research and secure comprehensive travel insurance with coverage for pre-existing conditions, including MG. Confirm that your insurance policy covers medical emergencies, hospital stays, and potential evacuation if needed. Understanding your insurance coverage provides peace of mind and ensures financial protection in unforeseen circumstances.

Assistive Devices

Consider the assistive devices you need for comfort and mobility when planning your travels. Consider whether it's more practical to bring your own mobility aids or rent them at your destination. If you plan to do a lot of walking or sightseeing, you might need a more supportive or robust device than you usually use. You can arrange for wheelchairs, walking aids, and other assistive devices in advance to ensure your travel experience meets your specific needs.

Medication Management

Ensure that you have an ample supply of necessary medications for the entire duration of your trip. If traveling internationally, check the regulations for carrying medications in your destination country, and carry a copy of your prescription. Discuss medication timing with your prescribing physician, especially if you will be changing time zones. Consider using a pill organizer to simplify medication management during your journey. (NOTE: If you take pyridostigmine, keep this medication in its original bottle as it is highly moisture-sensitive.)

Emergency Contact Information

Compile a list of emergency contact information, including your primary healthcare provider, MG specialist, and other medical providers involved in your care. It's also wise to have contact details for a close friend or family member who isn't traveling with you. Keep this information readily accessible on your phone and a printed copy in your wallet or bag to ensure quick communication and care coordination in unexpected situations.

By taking a proactive and informed approach to understanding your needs, consulting with healthcare professionals, and researching healthcare options at your destination, you can lay the groundwork for a smooth and enjoyable travel experience with Myasthenia Gravis. This strategic preparation enhances your overall well-being and ensures that you are equipped to navigate any potential challenges that may arise during your journey.

※

STRATEGIC REST BREAKS AND PACING THROUGHOUT THE JOURNEY

Traveling with MG requires a thoughtful approach to managing your energy levels. In this section, we'll explore the significance of strategic rest breaks and effective pacing strategies, empowering you to navigate your journey with resilience and well-being.

Plan Your Breaks

Understanding the importance of strategic breaks is fundamental to crafting a travel experience that aligns with your MG-specific needs. Breaks serve as essential intervals for rest, rejuvenation, and energy conservation. Whether you're embarking on a road trip, exploring a historical site, or navigating a bustling city, incorporating planned breaks into your itinerary is a proactive way to manage fatigue.

Consider the duration of your activities and intersperse them with adequate breaks. Factor in rest periods when planning your daily schedule, ensuring that you have moments of respite to recharge. Recognize that each individual's energy threshold varies, so tailor your breaks to suit your unique requirements.

Pacing Strategies

Balancing activity and rest is the key to optimizing energy levels throughout your journey. Pacing strategies involve a mindful approach to how you distribute your physical and mental exertion. It's a dynamic dance between engagement and recovery, allowing you to maintain a sustainable energy level.

Adjusting the pace of travel to your individual needs is paramount. Embrace a flexible mindset that accommodates the ebb and flow of energy inherent to MG. Listen to your body's cues and be responsive to signals of fatigue. If a planned activity feels strenuous, be prepared to modify or postpone it. Adopting a pacing strategy that aligns with your capabilities allows you to navigate your journey with greater ease and enjoyment.

Incorporating planned breaks and pacing yourself can turn travel from a source of stress into a truly enjoyable experience. By managing your energy levels throughout the trip, you'll not only make your travels more feasible but also more fulfilling and enriching. This way, you can explore the world with MG and truly enjoy every moment.

❄

GETTING FROM A TO B

Air Travel

Embarking on air travel with MG requires meticulous planning and thoughtful choices. In this section, we'll explore practical strategies to enhance your air travel experience, addressing the specific challenges that MG presents. From booking your flights to navigating the airport, let's ensure your journey is both feasible and enjoyable.

- **Booking Your Flight**: Choosing optimal flight times is crucial for a comfortable journey with MG. Consider your energy levels and natural sleep patterns when booking your flights. Opt for flights that match your peak energy periods to reduce fatigue. Additionally, avoid long flights or layovers that might worsen MG symptoms. When selecting seats, prioritize comfort and accessibility. If possible, choose seats with extra legroom near the front of the plane and close to the lavatory to make your trip more relaxed and convenient.
- **In-Flight Comfort:** Managing fatigue during long flights is essential for air travel with MG. Adjust your sleep schedule before your trip to help your body adapt to different time zones and reduce jet lag. Use relaxation techniques during the flight to ease the physical strain and reduce stress. Stay hydrated to counteract the dehydrating effects of high altitudes. Also, keep track of your medication schedule, considering time zone changes, to ensure consistent management of your MG symptoms.

- **Airport Navigation:** Navigating the airport with MG requires some extra planning. Wheelchair assistance can make moving through the airport more manageable and less stressful. Pre-boarding options are also helpful, letting you board the plane before other passengers so you have more time to get settled comfortably. Security screening accommodations are available to streamline the process and reduce potential challenges. Don't hesitate to communicate your needs to airline staff—they're there to help you throughout your journey.

By incorporating these suggestions into your air travel preparations, you can approach your journey with confidence and ease. Air travel with MG becomes a feasible and enjoyable experience when you make informed choices and prioritize your well-being. As you navigate the skies, remember that you have the tools and strategies to ensure a comfortable and pleasant journey.

Road Travel

I have fond memories of road trips, both as a kid and as an adult. However, MG poses its own unique challenges when it comes to extended car travel. As we explore road travel with MG, we'll cover practical strategies to make your car trips both comfortable and enjoyable.

- **Vehicle Selection:** Choosing the right vehicle is pivotal for a comfortable road trip. Consider vehicles with features that prioritize accessibility and ease. Automatic transmission is a game-changer, eliminating the need for frequent clutch engagement and reducing strain on your limbs. (While most vehicles sold in the United States have automatic transmission, manual transmission is still quite common in other countries. Consider this when selecting a vehicle.) Explore cars with adjustable seating options, allowing you to customize your position for optimal comfort during extended drives. Additionally, consider vehicles with a smooth suspension system to minimize the impact of road vibrations.

- **Strategic Rest Breaks:** Planning strategic rest breaks prevents fatigue during road trips. Schedule breaks at intervals that align with your energy levels, ensuring you have time to rest and rejuvenate. If your energy tends to wane later in the day, schedule more rest breaks during that time period. Identify suitable rest areas along your route, looking for locations with accessible facilities and amenities. Taking breaks helps manage MG-related fatigue and contributes to a more enjoyable and leisurely travel experience.

- **Accessible Facilities:** Before embarking on your journey, research and map out accessible facilities along your route. Identify rest areas and service stations with amenities designed for individuals with mobility challenges. Accessible facilities can provide the support and convenience needed to make your road trip more comfortable.

- **Comfortable Seating Solutions:** Enhance your in-car comfort with additional seating accessories. Consider investing in ergonomic cushions or lumbar support to alleviate discomfort during the drive. Experiment with different seat configurations and find the setup that provides optimal support for your back and neck.

- **Temperature Control:** Maintaining a comfortable temperature inside the car is crucial for managing MG symptoms. Ensure that your vehicle's climate control system is functioning well, and consider using seat covers that regulate temperature. Dress in layers, allowing you to adjust to changing temperatures without compromising comfort.

- **Plan Your Route:** Optimize your route planning by choosing roads with smoother surfaces and minimal roadwork. Use navigation apps that provide real-time updates on traffic conditions, helping you avoid congestion and potential stress triggers.

Integrating these strategies into your road travel preparations allows you to transform your journey into a comfortable and pleasurable experience. Car travel with MG becomes an opportunity to explore new destinations with confidence and ease, knowing that you have proactively addressed the unique considerations associated with MG.

Train Travel

Train travel is a great way to get around and is quite popular in Europe, Asia, and certain parts of North America (mainly the East and West coasts). However, rail travel presents a unique set of considerations for individuals with MG. In this section, we'll delve into practical strategies to ensure your train journey is not only accessible but also comfortable and enjoyable.

- **Choosing Train Services:** When selecting train services, prioritize those with accessibility features tailored to your needs. Look for stations with ramps and train cars that offer extra legroom, ensuring a more accommodating travel experience. Explore the available services to identify those that enhance accessibility, from boarding ramps to wheelchair-accessible facilities.

- **Booking Your Seat:** Booking seats strategically is critical to optimizing your comfort during the journey. Aim for seats with extra legroom and consider the proximity to essential facilities, such as the toilet and dining car, if applicable. This thoughtful approach to seat selection ensures you have the space and accessibility required for a relaxing train travel experience.
- **Caution When Moving:** If you have to get up to use the restroom or navigate to a different train car, be very cautious to maintain your balance and stability as the train is moving. Consider using an assistive device to help you keep your balance.
- **Onboard Comfort:** Making the most of your train journey involves adopting seating and relaxation strategies that align with MG-specific needs. Explore seating configurations to find the arrangement that provides optimal support for your back and neck. Consider bringing additional cushions or lumbar support to enhance your comfort during the trip. Stay hydrated and keep necessary snacks on hand to maintain energy levels throughout the journey.

As you embark on your train travel adventure, remember that thoughtful planning and strategic choices can significantly enhance your overall experience. By considering accessibility features, selecting comfortable seats, and adopting onboard strategies tailored to MG, you can relax and enjoy the scenic journey from the comfort of the train cabin. Train travel with MG becomes not just a mode of transportation but an opportunity to savor the journey with ease and accessibility.

❄

HOTEL ACCOMMODATIONS

Hotel stays are an integral part of travel, and thoughtful consideration of accommodations is crucial for individuals with MG. This section provides insights into maximizing comfort and accessibility during your hotel experience.

Accessible Room Features

Identifying and requesting hotel rooms with necessary accessibility features is a fundamental step in ensuring a comfortable stay. Look for rooms with features such as grab bars, accessible bathrooms, walk-in/roll-in showers, and wider doorways. Confirm that the hotel has designated accessible rooms and inquire about the specific features available in each room. (Not all "accessible" rooms are created equal.) Proximity to essential facilities, such as elevators and exits, further contributes to the convenience of your stay.

In addition to physical features, consider furniture placement within the room. Opt for a layout that allows for easy navigation and minimizes obstacles. Request room assignments that align with your mobility needs, promoting a smoother and more enjoyable stay.

Communication with Staff

Effective communication with hotel staff is key to addressing your specific needs and ensuring a tailored experience. Before your arrival, contact the hotel to communicate your requirements. This could include preferences for particular room features, additional pillows or bedding, or any other accommodations that contribute to your comfort. Clearly articulate your needs using specific and concise language. Request a written confirmation of your accommodation requests to ensure the hotel staff is aware and prepared for your arrival.

Upon check-in, take the opportunity to reiterate your needs and confirm that the accommodations are in place. Establishing open and clear communication sets the foundation for a positive hotel experience, allowing you to focus on enjoying your stay.

Navigating hotel accommodations with MG involves a proactive approach, from selecting accessible room features to fostering effective communication with the hotel staff. By considering these aspects, you can create a home away from home that prioritizes your comfort and accessibility, making your overall travel experience more enjoyable.

❄

NAVIGATING NON-DISABILITY-FRIENDLY SITES

Exploring historical sites and attractions that may not be inherently disability-friendly requires strategic planning and effective communication. In this section, we'll explore practical strategies for transforming potential challenges into opportunities for an enriching experience.

Research and Planning

The foundation for a successful visit to non-disability-friendly sites lies in thorough research and meticulous planning. Before your visit, invest time in understanding the layout and potential barriers of the site. Utilize online resources, travel forums, and accessibility guides to gather insights from others who have visited the location. Look for alternative routes, accessible entrances, and any available accommodations that might enhance your experience.

Identifying potential challenges allows you to plan your visit more effectively. Consider factors such as uneven terrain, staircases, or limited seating areas. By anticipating these challenges, you can develop strategies to navigate the site more comfortably. Explore the availability of guided tours or assistance services that may provide additional support.

Communication with Staff at Sites

Prior to your visit, reach out to the site's management or visitor services to discuss your specific accessibility requirements. Clearly articulate your needs and inquire about any accommodations they may offer. This proactive communication allows staff to prepare for your visit, making necessary arrangements to enhance accessibility.

During your visit, maintain open and respectful communication with site staff. If you encounter unexpected challenges, seek assistance promptly. Many historical sites have staff members dedicated to visitor services who can provide guidance and support. Don't hesitate to advocate for reasonable accommodations that may enhance your ability to explore and enjoy the site.

By adopting a proactive approach to research, planning, and effective communication, you can navigate non-disability-friendly sites with greater confidence. A bit of strategic planning will ensure that your travel experiences are not limited by physical barriers but enriched by the wealth of cultural and historical wonders.

❄

EMERGENCY PREPAREDNESS AND CONTINGENCY PLANS

Navigating the unexpected is an integral aspect of travel, and proactive emergency preparedness is paramount for individuals with

MG. In this section, we'll discuss comprehensive strategies for ensuring your well-being in unforeseen circumstances.

Medication Management

Ensuring a seamless continuation of your medication regimen is a cornerstone of emergency preparedness. Begin by organizing and packing an ample supply of your necessary medications for the entire duration of your journey. Consider factors such as time zone changes and potential delays to ensure you have a buffer supply.

In addition to packing medications, create a comprehensive medical information card. This card should include essential details such as your medical conditions, prescribed medications, dosage instructions, and any allergies. It should also include emergency contact information for both local and home contacts. Keep this card with you at all times, whether in your wallet or a designated travel pouch, for quick accessibility.

Navigating Unforeseen Challenges

Strategies for handling unexpected situations or MG exacerbations are crucial components of your contingency plans. Familiarize yourself with local medical facilities and emergency services at your travel destination. Research nearby hospitals, clinics, and pharmacies, noting their accessibility and available services.

Have a clear plan in place in case of an MG exacerbation or unforeseen challenge. Communicate your condition promptly to travel companions, and if needed, seek assistance from local emergency services. If applicable, carry a list of phrases in the local language that convey essential information about your condition and the assistance required.

Understanding the layout of your accommodation, including evacuation routes, emergency exits, and accessible facilities, contributes to a comprehensive contingency plan. Share your emergency plan with travel companions, ensuring they know the steps to take in case of unforeseen challenges.

By meticulously preparing for medication management and developing strategies for navigating unforeseen challenges, you strengthen your ability to respond effectively to any emergencies that may arise. This proactive approach enhances your safety during travel and instills confidence, allowing you to focus on thoroughly enjoying your travel experience.

❄

Traveling with MG requires significant planning and adjustments, but the opportunity to explore new places and cultures is well worth it. With careful planning and flexibility, travel with MG can be manageable and deeply fulfilling. Successful travel with MG is a fusion of careful planning, effective communication, resilience, and a positive attitude. Prioritize your well-being, embrace the strategies outlined in this chapter, and approach your adventures with the spirit of enjoyment.

Safe travels!

TAKE-HOME POINTS

1. **Plan ahead**: Understand your MG symptoms and consult with healthcare providers before travel to manage medications and anticipate needs.
2. **Prioritize comfort and accessibility**: Choose travel options, accommodations, and activities that support your physical well-being and minimize stress.
3. **Embrace pacing and breaks**: Strategically schedule rest

periods to manage fatigue and optimize energy levels throughout your journey.

4. **Communicate your needs**: Advocate for yourself by informing airline and hotel staff about your condition and necessary accommodations.

5. **Be prepared for emergencies**: Carry emergency contact information, medications, and a medical information card to respond effectively to unexpected situations.

Chapter 8

Asking for Help

LET'S TALK ABOUT SOMETHING THAT MANY OF US FIND challenging: asking for help. I get it—I struggle with it too. There have been countless times when I've stubbornly plodded along with a task, convinced that I could handle it on my own, only to have my husband gently inquire, "Are you going to ask me for help with that?" It's a question that always gives me pause because it touches on a more profound truth: asking for help can feel like admitting defeat, like acknowledging that we're not as strong or independent as we'd like to be. But here's the thing: managing Myasthenia Gravis (MG) is tough, and none of us can do it alone. We're navigating a condition that profoundly impacts our daily lives, from the simplest tasks to the most significant challenges. And while it's natural to want to maintain a sense of autonomy and self-sufficiency, the reality is that there are times when we need assistance. Recognizing when we need help and being willing to ask for it is a sign of strength, not weakness. It's a testament to our resilience and our willingness to do whatever it takes to manage our health and well-being.

In this chapter, we will delve into the personal struggles associated with asking for help while also highlighting the importance of seeking assistance in managing MG and maintaining our quality of life. We'll explore the different forms that help can take, from leaning on our loved ones to accessing community resources and professional services. Most importantly, we'll learn that asking for help isn't a sign of weakness—it's a necessary part of living with MG and something we can do together every step of the way.

You've already taken a step in getting help for your MG by reading this book. So, let's tackle this together.

❄

ASKING FOR HELP FROM FAMILY AND FRIENDS

Living with MG often requires leaning on a support network for assistance with various tasks. From household chores to running errands, there are many areas where individuals with MG may need help from family, friends, and the community. However, it's essential to acknowledge that everyone's personal, family, and community situation differs. While some people may have a robust support network readily available, others may have more limited resources to rely on. Similarly, family dynamics and relationships can vary greatly, influencing the ease or difficulty of asking for help. Community resources and accessibility may also differ depending on location and available services.

Household chores, such as cleaning, laundry, and gardening, can become physically demanding and exhausting for someone with MG. Asking for help with these tasks can lighten the load and prevent overexertion. Similarly, meal preparation can be challenging, especially when fatigue sets in, making it difficult to stand for long periods or manage heavy pots and pans. Seeking assistance with meal prep can ensure that nutritious meals are still enjoyed without the added strain and stress. Individuals with MG may also require assistance running errands and generally getting around, whether driving or using public transportation. Having someone to assist with driving or accompanying you can make daily tasks more manageable, such as grocery shopping, attending appointments, or getting to social engagements.

Given the variability of individual circumstances, open communication is vital when asking for help from loved ones. It's important to be honest about your limitations and needs while also respecting their boundaries and availability. Setting clear expectations and discussing how they can best support you can help prevent misunderstandings and ensure that assistance is provided in a helpful and meaningful way. Additionally, expressing gratitude for the support you receive is essential. Letting your loved ones know how much their help means to you and acknowledging their efforts can strengthen your relationships and foster a sense of mutual support and appreciation.

Asking for help from family, friends, and the community is vital to managing MG. While everyone's personal, family, and community situation may differ, building a solid support network and communicating openly about your needs can enhance your quality of life and allow you to navigate the challenges of living with MG more effectively.

PRO TIP: *Shift your mindset from guilt to gratitude. When asking for help, it is common to feel guilty, as if it's an imposition. But remember that those who love you want to help you. So, think "grateful" instead of "guilty." In conversation, instead of "I'm sorry for troubling you," try, "Thank you for helping me."*

❄

HIRING HELP (BUDGET PERMITTING)

Living with MG often entails managing a range of household tasks that can become challenging due to MG-related limitations. When daily chores start to feel overwhelming, seeking professional help can be a practical solution to lighten the load and ensure essential tasks are completed without risking overexertion. Depending on your personal financial situation, consider one or more of the following:

- **Housekeeping Services**: Consider enlisting the help of a professional housekeeping service to manage regular household chores. These services typically offer a range of cleaning options, including dusting, vacuuming, mopping floors, and cleaning bathrooms and kitchens. Hiring a housekeeper can ensure that your home remains clean and organized without requiring you to expend precious energy on these tasks.
- **Meal Preparation Services**: Cooking meals can be particularly challenging for individuals with MG, especially during periods of fatigue or weakness. Using a meal preparation service or hiring someone to help with cooking can alleviate the stress of planning and cooking meals while ensuring you still enjoy nutritious and delicious food. Many meal preparation services offer customized meal plans to accommodate dietary restrictions and preferences, providing convenient and healthy meal options tailored to your needs.
- **Landscaping and Yard Work**: Outdoor maintenance tasks such as mowing the lawn, trimming hedges, and tending to flower beds can quickly become exhausting for individuals with MG. Working outside in the heat can be extremely difficult and potentially dangerous, depending on where you live and the time of year. Hiring a landscaping

or yard work service can help maintain your outdoor space without requiring you to exert yourself physically. These professionals can handle tasks such as lawn mowing, pruning, weeding, and seasonal cleanup, allowing you to enjoy your outdoor environment without the strain.

- **Errand and Shopping Services**: Running errands and grocery shopping can be time-consuming and physically demanding for individuals with MG. Consider hiring an errand or shopping service to take care of these tasks on your behalf. These services can handle everything from picking up prescriptions and dry cleaning to grocery shopping and meal delivery, saving you time and energy while ensuring that your essential needs are met.

- **In-Home Aides**: For individuals with more extensive care needs, hiring an in-home aide can provide invaluable support with personal care, mobility assistance, and daily activities. In-home aides can assist with tasks such as bathing, dressing, medication management, and companionship, allowing you to maintain your independence and quality of life at home. Additionally, they can provide respite care for family caregivers, offering much-needed relief and support.

When considering hiring professional help, it's essential to assess your individual needs and budget accordingly. Research local service providers to compare rates, services offered, and customer reviews. Additionally, explore potential funding options, such as government assistance programs or insurance coverage, to help offset the costs of hiring professional assistance. By investing in professional help, you can alleviate the physical strain and stress associated with managing household tasks while living with MG, allowing you to focus on activities that bring you joy and fulfillment.

❄

SEEKING ASSISTANCE IN THE COMMUNITY

Navigating public settings with MG can present unique challenges, but practical solutions are available to help make tasks more manageable. When you find yourself in places like grocery stores or shopping malls, consider utilizing motorized scooters provided by these establishments. These scooters offer mobility assistance, allowing you to conserve your energy and reduce physical strain while navigating large spaces. Take advantage of these resources to ensure you have the stamina to complete your errands and enjoy your outing without feeling exhausted.

Additionally, don't hesitate to request assistance from store staff when faced with challenging tasks such as reaching high shelves or lifting heavy objects. Many store employees are trained to assist customers with disabilities. And even if they are not, they are typically more than willing to lend a helping hand if asked. Whether grabbing items from a high shelf or carrying a heavy item to your car, don't hesitate to ask for assistance when needed. Remember, your well-being is essential, and seeking help when necessary is a proactive step toward managing your MG effectively.

It's understandable to feel hesitant or embarrassed about asking for help in public places, but it's essential to overcome these feelings to prioritize your comfort and safety. Consider practicing assertive communication techniques and preparing a brief explanation of your condition and the type of assistance you require (if you feel comfortable doing so). Remember, you're not alone in facing these challenges. Many individuals with MG encounter similar obstacles when out and about, and there's no shame in asking for help to ensure a smooth and enjoyable experience. By embracing the support available and advocating for your needs, you can confidently navigate public settings and maintain your independence while managing your MG effectively.

❄

GOVERNMENT AND COMMUNITY PROGRAMS

Living with MG often necessitates tapping into a variety of government and community support programs tailored to assist individuals with disabilities. These programs offer valuable resources and accommodations to alleviate the challenges associated with MG and enhance your overall quality of life.

- **Disabled Parking Permits**: Individuals with MG may have difficulty walking long distances or standing for extended periods, making it challenging to find suitable parking spots. Disabled parking permits provide access to designated parking spaces closer to buildings and facilities, making outings more accessible and manageable. To apply for a disabled parking permit, contact your local Department of Motor Vehicles (DMV) or relevant government agency. Provide documentation of necessity from your medical provider and any other required information to qualify for the permit.
- **Airport Assistance Services**: Traveling with MG can present unique challenges, especially when navigating busy airports and managing luggage. Many airports offer assistance services for travelers with disabilities, including wheelchair assistance, pre-boarding options, and assistance with navigating security checkpoints. To access these services, contact your airline or the airport directly before your travel date. Inform them of your specific

needs due to MG and request assistance accordingly. Airport staff are trained to provide support and accommodations to ensure a smoother travel experience for individuals with disabilities.

- **Accessible Transportation Services**: Many communities offer accessible transportation services for individuals with disabilities who may have difficulty driving or using traditional public transit options. These services may include paratransit services, wheelchair-accessible vans, and specialized transportation programs. Contact your local transit authority or disability services office to inquire about available transportation options in your area.

- **Financial Assistance Programs**: Various financial assistance programs are available to individuals with disabilities to help cover essential expenses such as housing, utilities, and medical costs. Examples of such programs in the United States include Supplemental Security Income (SSI), Social Security Disability Insurance (SSDI), and Medicaid. Eligibility criteria and application processes vary, so it's essential to research and contact the relevant government agencies or advocacy organizations for guidance.

- **Assistive Technology Programs**: Assistive technology can significantly enhance independence and accessibility for individuals with disabilities. Many government and nonprofit organizations offer programs to help individuals acquire assistive devices such as wheelchairs, mobility aids, communication devices, and adaptive computer equipment. Explore resources available from organizations like the Assistive Technology Act Program in the United States and country, state, or region-specific assistive technology programs relevant to where you live.

- **Vocational Rehabilitation Services**: Vocational rehabilitation programs help individuals with disabilities prepare for, obtain, and maintain employment. These programs offer a range of services, including vocational counseling, job training, job placement assistance, and workplace accommodations. In the United States, contact your state's vocational rehabilitation agency or the Department of Labor's Office of Disability Employment Policy (ODEP) to learn more about available services and eligibility requirements.
- **Home Modification Assistance**: Various programs offer financial assistance for home modifications for individuals with disabilities who require improvements to their living environment to improve accessibility and safety. These modifications may include installing ramps, grab bars, stairlifts, and accessible bathroom fixtures. Explore resources provided by housing agencies, nonprofit organizations, and disability advocacy groups to find assistance with home modifications.

By exploring these and other government and community support programs, individuals with MG can access valuable resources and accommodations to help navigate daily life with greater ease and independence. Take proactive steps to research available programs, determine eligibility criteria, and apply for the assistance you need to enhance your quality of life while living with MG.

❋

SEEKING PROFESSIONAL HELP

Managing the challenges of living with MG often requires the expertise and support of various healthcare professionals who specialize in addressing the unique needs of individuals with chronic illnesses. Seeking professional help can play a crucial role in improving overall quality of life and enhancing the management of MG-related symptoms. When seeking help in the medical system, it's easy to stop with the physician. However, there is a wide range of healthcare providers who can be instrumental in helping people with MG learn to move better, conserve energy, and generally have a better quality of life.

- **Physical Therapy (PT)**: Physical therapists (or physiotherapists) are instrumental in helping individuals with MG optimize movement, mobility, and muscle strength. As a PT myself, I recognize that I might be accused of bias here. However, PTs are universally recognized as movement experts. PTs can address weakness, improve balance and coordination, and enhance overall physical function through tailored exercise programs, neuromuscular retraining techniques, and assistive devices. Additionally, they can provide education on energy conservation strategies and safe exercise practices to help individuals with MG manage their symptoms effectively.
- **Occupational Therapy (OT)**: Occupational therapists specialize in helping individuals with MG maintain independence and participate in meaningful daily activities. They can assess functional abilities, recommend adaptive equipment and assistive devices, and provide training in energy conservation techniques to conserve energy and minimize fatigue. OTs also offer guidance on modifying the home environment to improve accessibility and safety, ensuring that individuals with MG can engage in daily tasks more comfortably and efficiently.

- **Speech-Language Pathology (SLP)**: Speech-language pathologists, also called speech therapists, play a vital role in addressing communication and swallowing difficulties commonly experienced by individuals with MG. They can provide specialized interventions to improve speech clarity, articulation, and vocal strength, as well as techniques to enhance swallowing function and prevent aspiration. SLPs may also offer dietary recommendations and strategies to manage dysphagia (difficulty swallowing), ensuring that individuals with MG can maintain adequate nutrition and hydration safely.
- **Respiratory Therapy (RT)**: Respiratory therapists specialize in evaluating and treating respiratory disorders, including respiratory muscle weakness and compromised lung function associated with MG. They can provide respiratory assessments, breathing exercises, and airway clearance techniques to optimize lung function and improve respiratory efficiency. RTs may also recommend non-invasive ventilation devices, such as bilevel-positive airway pressure (BiPAP) machines, to support breathing and alleviate respiratory symptoms in individuals with MG.
- **Psychotherapy or Counseling**: In addition to outpatient rehabilitation services, seeking counseling or psychotherapy can be beneficial for individuals with MG in addressing emotional challenges and coping with the psychological impact of living with a chronic illness. Counseling sessions can provide a supportive space to explore feelings of depression, anxiety, stress, and grief associated with MG and develop coping strategies to enhance emotional well-being and resilience.

By seeking professional help from a multidisciplinary team of healthcare professionals, individuals with MG can access comprehensive support and tailored interventions to address their unique needs and improve their overall quality of life. Working collaboratively with these professionals can empower individuals with MG to effectively manage their symptoms, enhance independence, and achieve their personal goals despite the challenges posed by the condition.

※

It's crucial to recognize that asking for help is not a sign of weakness but rather a strength in managing MG and maintaining overall well-being. Asking for help can be challenging, and it's essential to acknowledge and address any barriers or hesitations that may exist. By overcoming these barriers and embracing the support available, individuals with MG can enhance their quality of life and better manage their symptoms.

Remember, you are not alone in your journey with MG. Reach out to your support network, whether it's for assistance with daily tasks, accessing community resources, or seeking professional help from healthcare providers. Together, we can navigate the challenges of MG and empower ourselves to live fulfilling and meaningful lives despite the obstacles we may face.

Chapter 9

In Case of Emergency

EMERGENCIES HAPPEN. WHILE THERE IS A LOT WE CAN DO to prevent or mitigate, the truth is that emergencies can (and sometimes do) still happen. Despite strictly adhering to a healthy routine of medication, energy conservation strategies, healthy activity, and a mindful diet and eating habits, a myasthenic crisis is still a possibility. (Though solid management of MG should significantly reduce this risk.) Other medical emergencies can happen, too, and it's important to be prepared. So, while this topic is not necessarily related to energy conservation like the rest of the book, I would be remiss not covering how to handle an emergency with Myasthenia Gravis (MG).

First things first, what is a myasthenic crisis? In the simplest of terms, a myasthenic crisis occurs when the muscles of respiration, chiefly the diaphragm, become fatigued to the point where it is extremely difficult to breathe, and the diaphragm is unable to recover sufficiently.[1] While diaphragm fatigue is more common, it is also

---

1. Wendell, L. C., & Levine, J. M. (2011). Myasthenic Crisis. *The Neurohospitalist*, *1*(1), 16-22. https://doi.org/10.1177/1941875210382918

possible to have an upper airway restriction caused by weakened laryngeal muscles (also called "vocal cord paralysis"). I mention this because, though it is less common, it is still a cause of respiratory distress in MG and is often overlooked or mistaken for asthma.[2] Regardless of the source of breathing difficulty, it is an emergency, under no uncertain terms, requiring medical attention.

Every case of myasthenic crisis looks different. I have lived with this disease for years, I have treated many cases of MG, and I have studied the disorder at length. However, even I had trouble recognizing the signs when I went into a myasthenic crisis myself.

It was my birthday. (Of course it was...) I had worked a long day and had enjoyed a nice dinner at home with my family. As I put the kids to bed that night, I felt like I was dragging more than usual. *Oh well*, I thought to myself, *I must have overdone it today. No big deal.*

Wrong.

The next day, I woke up feeling worse—like I hadn't slept at all. My vision was doubled, my right eyelid was half closed, and I choked on my morning coffee. Walking across the room felt like walking waist-deep through mud. I took the day off of work and rested, but I didn't improve much. By the evening, I was having trouble breathing with just the short walk from my bed to the bathroom. (NOTE: In retrospect, this is where I probably should have gone to the ER or, at a minimum, called my neurologist's answering service, but I was stubborn. So please, do as I say, not as I did.)

By three o'clock in the morning, I was having trouble breathing at rest in a recliner. Did I go to the ER then? I should have! But no, I didn't. Foolishly, I was too worried about waking my household, disrupting our schedule, finding childcare, and generally being a bother. So, I waited until the morning.

---

2. Ping-Hung Kuo and Pi-Chuan Fan (2012). Respiratory Care for Myasthenic Crisis, A Look into Myasthenia Gravis, Dr. Joseph A. Pruitt (Ed.), ISBN: 978-953-307-821-2, InTech, Available from: http://www.intechopen.com/books/a-look-into-myasthenia-gravis/respiratory-care-for-myasthenic-crisis

After my husband and I dropped the kids off at daycare, he drove me to the emergency room. Thankfully, it wasn't busy first thing on a Friday morning. I thought I would be in and out quickly after a few tests, a chest X-ray, and a prescription. I thought I might have a respiratory infection that was making my MG flare up.

Wrong again.

In the short time it took me to crutch from the car to the check-in desk (on a hot, sticky, humid summer morning in South Carolina), my breathing worsened rapidly, and I collapsed at the desk. Full-blown MG crisis.

To make a long story short, I spent the next week in the intensive care unit on some degree of ventilatory support, receiving aggressive intravenous immunoglobulin (IVIG) treatment.

It took me a month until I was ready to return to work on a limited basis and six months of physical therapy until my strength and mobility were back to normal.

The moral of this story: take breathing difficulties in MG seriously and seek help sooner rather than later.

❄

WHAT TO LOOK OUT FOR: SIGNS OF AN IMPENDING MYASTHENIC CRISIS

Signs of a myasthenic crisis can be subtle at first, but they quickly escalate into a medical emergency that requires immediate attention. As someone who has experienced this myself, I want to emphasize how important it is to be vigilant and aware of the potential warning signs of a crisis. Here's what to look out for:

- **Breathing difficulties**: This is the hallmark sign of a myasthenic crisis. You may notice shortness of breath at rest or during mild activity. Breathing may become labored, and you might struggle to take deep breaths. If you find yourself struggling to breathe while sitting down, lying down, or doing simple tasks, you need to seek medical help immediately.

- **Difficulty swallowing**: Dysphagia, or difficulty swallowing, is another critical symptom. You may notice trouble chewing food, choking on liquids, or coughing while eating or drinking. This can be a sign that your respiratory and swallowing muscles are compromised.
- **Speech changes**: A crisis can affect the muscles involved in speaking, leading to slurred or nasal speech. Your voice might sound weaker, raspy, or generally different from your usual tone.
- **Visual changes**: Double vision or drooping eyelids can occur as the muscles around your eyes become fatigued. This can impair your vision and make it difficult to see clearly.
- **Generalized weakness**: You may experience overall muscle weakness that can impact your ability to perform routine activities. If your arms and legs feel heavier than usual, or you struggle to perform movements that were once easy, this could be a sign of a crisis.

It's crucial to recognize these symptoms as they can rapidly worsen. If you experience any of these signs, and they do not adequately respond to rest, do not wait for them to resolve on their own. Seek medical attention immediately. Being proactive can save your life and prevent the crisis from escalating further. Keep in mind that a crisis can unfold differently for everyone, so pay attention to any changes in your body, and don't hesitate to call for help if you suspect a myasthenic crisis is occurring.

❄

PLAN AHEAD: DEVELOP AN EMERGENCY ACTION PLAN

Developing an emergency management plan with your neurologist is one of the most critical steps you can take to prepare for potential emergencies related to MG. Collaborating with your neurologist allows you to create a personalized plan that suits your specific needs and circumstances. This plan can help guide you and your loved ones through a crisis situation, minimizing uncertainty and ensuring you receive timely and appropriate care.

To create an effective emergency management plan, start by identifying early warning signs and the actions you should take when they occur. These signs can vary depending on the individual, but common indicators of a myasthenic crisis include increased muscle weakness, difficulty swallowing, and shortness of breath. Your neurologist can help you recognize these warning signs and outline the steps you should take if you experience them.

Next, discuss potential treatments or interventions that might be necessary during a crisis. This may include ventilatory support and treatment options like intravenous immunoglobulin (IVIG) or plasmapheresis, which can help stabilize your condition. Knowing these treatment possibilities in advance can help you and your loved ones better understand what to expect and how to respond during a crisis.

It's also essential to have a clear plan for when to seek medical attention. Your neurologist can help you establish guidelines for when to go to the emergency room or call an ambulance. This plan should include information on local emergency departments, the contact information for your neurologist or other specialists, and any specific instructions regarding your care.

Finally, ensure that your emergency management plan includes options for different scenarios, such as what to do if you are alone during a crisis or traveling away from home. Discussing these possibilities with your neurologist and having a plan in place will provide peace of mind and a sense of control in an emergency.

※

AT-HOME BREATHING ASSESSMENTS

Monitoring your respiratory function at home is vital to managing MG and can provide valuable insights into your overall health. At-home breathing assessments are essential for detecting changes in respiratory strength and identifying signs of weakness or fatigue early on. By regularly performing tests such as the Negative Inspiratory Force (NIF) test, spirometry, and the Single Breath Count Test (SBCT), you can proactively monitor your lung function and identify potential issues before they escalate. Recognizing changes in your respiratory capacity can also help you determine when it may be necessary to seek emergency medical attention.

Objective breathing assessments, such as the Negative Inspiratory Force (NIF) test and spirometry, can provide valuable insights into lung function and respiratory health for individuals living with MG. The NIF test measures the strength of the muscles involved in inhaling, while spirometry assesses lung capacity and airflow. These assessments are essential because changes in respiratory function can indicate worsening symptoms or the onset of a myasthenic crisis.

However, while portable, easy-to-use devices are available for these tests, not everyone has access to specialized equipment like spirometers at home. That's where the Single Breath Count Test (SBCT) comes in handy. This simple yet effective test requires no equipment and can be performed anywhere, anytime. The SBCT essentially measures the amount of air a person can inhale and utilize effectively in a single breath, offering valuable insights into their respiratory function.

To perform the SBCT, take a deep breath and count out loud at a rate of 120 beats per minute (bpm) until you run out of air. This pace is equivalent to a normalized counting rate and can be compared to popular songs with a tempo of 120 bpm, such as "Don't Stop Believin'" by Journey or "Girls Just Wanna Have Fun" by Cyndi Lauper. If songs aren't quite your thing, try a metronome app set to 120 bpm. (Or go old school and use an actual metronome if you happen to have one lying around.) Whichever method you choose, counting at 120 bpm ensures an accurate and consistent assessment of your breath count.

Regularly performing the SBCT allows you to track changes in your respiratory function and detect any abnormalities early on without requiring specialized equipment. While not an officially recognized measure with normative data at the time of this writing, studies demonstrate that results from the SBCT, when performed correctly, correlate with standardized lung function tests such as forced vital capacity (FVC), forced expiratory volume (FEV1), and negative inspiratory force (NIF)[3]. Additionally, the SBCT has been found to accurately predict the need for respiratory support or mechanical ventilation in patients with neuromuscular disorders, including MG.[4] If you notice a significant decrease in your breath count or experience difficulty breathing during the test, it may indicate the need for further evaluation by a healthcare professional.

Still need help knowing how fast 120 bpm is? These songs can serve as a reference for maintaining the correct counting pace during the Single Breath Count exercise.

3. Elsheikh, B., Arnold, W. D., Gharibshahi, S., Reynolds, J., Freimer, M., & Kissel, J. T. (2016). Correlation of single-breath count test and neck flexor muscle strength with spirometry in myasthenia gravis. *Muscle & Nerve, 53*(1), 134. https://doi.org/10.1002/mus.24929
4. Bhandari, S. K., Bist, A., & Ghimire, A. (2024). Single breath count test and its applications in clinical practice: A systematic review. *Annals of Medicine and Surgery, 86*(4), 2130-2136. https://doi.org/10.1097/MS9.0000000000001853

Popular Songs with a Tempo of 120 bpm:

- "I Will Survive" by Gloria Gaynor
- "1999" by Prince
- "Wouldn't It Be Nice" by The Beach Boys
- "Poker Face" by Lady Gaga
- "I Heard It Through the Grapevine" by Creedence Clearwater Revival
- "Call Me Maybe" by Carly Rae Jepsen
- "Uptown Funk" by Mark Ronson feat. Bruno Mars
- "C is for Cookie" by Cookie Monster ("Sesame Street")

❄

IT'S GO TIME: WHAT TO PACK IN YOUR ER GO-BAG

Preparing for a potential emergency room or hospital trip is crucial for individuals with MG. When an emergency arises, having a go-bag ready can save precious time and provide you with the necessary items for a smooth and efficient experience at the hospital. Here's a comprehensive list of what to pack in your go-bag:

- **Medications**: Pack a supply of your current prescriptions, including any medications you take for MG or other conditions. It's important to have a list of your medications with dosages and schedules written down for reference, as well as an extra set of prescriptions in case you need them during a more extended hospital stay.
- **Medical Records**: Keep a copy of your medical history, including your diagnosis, surgeries, and any known

allergies. Include a record of your current treatment plan and any recent test results. This information can help medical personnel understand your condition and provide you with the proper care.

- **Contact Information**: Have a list of emergency contacts, including family members and healthcare providers. Include contact information for your neurologist and primary care provider, as well as the contact details of anyone who should be notified in case of emergency.
- **Advance Directives and Healthcare Proxy**: If you have any advance directives or healthcare proxies, pack a copy of these documents in your go-bag. This ensures that your medical decisions are honored and your healthcare wishes are known.
- **Identification and Insurance Information**: Bring your identification and insurance cards. These are essential for hospital admissions and can help ensure you receive the necessary care without unnecessary delays.
- **Respiratory Support Devices**: If you use a portable ventilator, BiPAP machine, or other respiratory support device, pack it along with extra supplies such as tubing, filters, and batteries (if applicable). Having these items on hand can be critical in a myasthenic crisis.
- **Personal Care Items**: Bring a few comfortable changes of clothes, including sleepwear and undergarments. Also, pack toiletries such as a toothbrush, toothpaste, deodorant, baby wipes, hand sanitizer, and any other items that make you feel more comfortable and at home.
- **Mobile Phone and Charger**: Your mobile phone is essential for staying connected with loved ones and your medical team. Pack a charger to ensure your phone remains charged throughout your hospital stay.

- **Snacks and Drinks**: Depending on your condition and dietary restrictions, pack a few snacks and drinks that you know you can tolerate. This can help tide you over while waiting for treatment and during your hospital stay. (Note: When you get to the ER, do not eat or drink anything until cleared by your medical team. Food or drink may interfere with certain tests and procedures.)
- **Entertainment and Comfort Items**: Bring items that will help you pass the time and provide comfort, such as a book, magazine, or music player. A small blanket or pillow from home can also make your hospital stay more comfortable.

Being prepared with a well-stocked go-bag can help alleviate stress during a medical emergency and ensure you have everything you need for your hospital visit. Review your go-bag regularly to make sure it remains up to date with your current needs and medications. By taking these proactive steps, you can be better equipped to handle an unexpected trip to the emergency room or hospital.

❄

RESOURCES FOR EMERGENCY RESPONDERS WORKING WITH MG

Due to the unique challenges posed by MG, emergencies require a specialized approach. Fortunately, valuable online resources are available to help emergency responders effectively manage MG emergencies. These resources offer educational materials, guidelines, and tools specifically tailored to the needs of individuals living with MG.

While many organizations and websites provide extremely

helpful information and resources for MG, I will focus on the resources available through the Myasthenia Gravis Foundation of America (MGFA). (NOTE: I am neither sponsored by nor directly affiliated with the MGFA, and I am not actively promoting them in this book. I chose to reference the resources available from the MGFA because they are the ones I am most familiar with and use. Many comparable resources are available from other national, international, and commercial MG organizations. It doesn't matter to me whose resources you choose to use. What matters to me is that you gather your resources and have them ready should you need them.)

Websites such as the MGFA, located at www.myasthenia.org, provide a wealth of knowledge about the condition, its symptoms, treatments, and emergency management strategies. The MGFA has a handout about MG emergency management written specifically for first responders, as well as a separate document for patients and caregivers. These resources are valuable reference tools, allowing emergency responders to quickly access relevant information when responding to MG-related emergencies. Notably, a list of contraindicated and precautionary medications in MG is available to help prevent the administration of medication that may be harmful to someone with MG. This is a great resource to have on hand if you have to visit the emergency room. (I always keep several copies printed out in my go-bag.) Also, a guide for respiratory assessment in MG is helpful, as respiratory distress and breathing difficulties present differently in MG compared with other medical conditions and can easily be overlooked.

Effective communication is essential in emergency situations involving individuals with MG. Online resources offer tools and guidelines for facilitating communication between emergency responders and MG patients. These tools include communication cards, medical alert bracelets, and other resources designed to help emergency responders understand and accommodate the specific needs of individuals with MG during emergencies.

By utilizing these online resources, emergency responders can enhance their knowledge, skills, and preparedness in managing MG emergencies, ultimately ensuring the best possible outcomes for individuals living with the condition.

❄

EMERGENCY ROOM VISITS FOR NON-MG CONDITIONS

Even though individuals with MG may primarily associate emergency room visits with myasthenic crises, it's crucial to seek emergency care for other conditions as well, such as falls, illnesses, accidents, or other unexpected events. Healthcare providers must be aware of your MG diagnosis during these situations, as it can impact treatment decisions. Always carry a medical alert card or bracelet with details about your MG diagnosis, current medications, known allergies, and emergency contact information. This ensures emergency room staff can deliver appropriate care tailored to your needs. Additionally, having an emergency management plan with contact information for your healthcare providers and loved ones can streamline communication and decision-making. By proactively preparing for emergency room visits, you can receive the care you need and minimize potential complications.

❄

BOTTOM LINE

Communication plays a vital role in emergency preparedness. As someone with MG, it is essential to communicate openly and regularly with your healthcare providers, loved ones, and emergency responders about your condition, symptoms, and emergency management plans. By fostering open lines of communication, you ensure that everyone involved in your care is well-informed and prepared to respond appropriately in an emergency.

Empowering yourself with the knowledge and tools to handle a crisis confidently and effectively is paramount. Through education, preparation, and proactive communication, you can navigate MG-related emergencies with confidence and resilience. By working together with healthcare providers, loved ones, and emergency responders, you can optimize your safety and well-being, even in challenging circumstances.

And to answer the question, "Should I go to the ER...?"

If you think you should, you should.

Chapter 10

Grace, Compassion, and Self Care

LIVING WITH MYASTHENIA GRAVIS (MG) CAN FEEL LIKE tackling a mountain every day. The tiredness that never leaves, the muscles that won't listen, and all those other tricky symptoms can turn even easy tasks into tough challenges. As someone with both personal and professional experience with MG, I understand the struggles that come with this condition. However, I have also learned the importance of practicing grace, compassion, and self-care in order to cope and thrive while living with MG. This is undoubtedly the most important thing we can do for ourselves.

In this final chapter, I want to focus on the importance of taking care of oneself, especially when living with a chronic condition like MG. As discussed throughout this book, energy conservation skills are crucial for managing MG. But self-care goes far beyond simply conserving energy. It involves showing yourself kindness, patience, and understanding. It means making your physical and mental well-being a priority. It means giving yourself the grace to navigate through the challenges of MG while still finding joy and purpose in life.

❄

Show Yourself Grace

The first step towards practicing self-care and compassion is to show yourself grace.

Yes, you.

What does this mean exactly? To me, showing grace means being kind and forgiving towards yourself, especially when facing challenges and limitations due to MG. It means accepting that you may not be able to do everything you used to do before, and that's okay. It means acknowledging your strengths and accomplishments, no matter how small they may seem.

As someone living with MG, I have learned the importance of showing myself grace on a daily basis. Some days, my symptoms may be more severe, and I may not be able to do as much as I would like. On those days, instead of getting frustrated and beating myself up, I remind myself that it's okay to take a break and rest. I remind myself that I am doing the best I can, and that's enough.

It's important to remember that MG is a chronic condition that can sometimes be unpredictable. (Understatement of the year!?) There may be days when you feel great and can do everything you want, and there may be days when your symptoms flare up and make it difficult to even get out of bed. It's crucial to have patience and understanding with yourself on those difficult days. Show yourself grace and know that tomorrow is a new day to start fresh.

Be Compassionate Towards Yourself

Living with a chronic condition like MG can also take a toll on your mental and emotional well-being. It's not uncommon to feel frustrated, anxious, or even depressed while managing this condition.

That's why it's essential to be compassionate towards yourself and acknowledge the emotional side of living with MG.

Self-compassion means recognizing and accepting your feelings and emotions without judgment. It means allowing yourself to feel whatever you are feeling and giving yourself the space to process those emotions. It's also about being understanding and gentle with yourself, especially when facing challenging situations.

As someone who has experienced the emotional rollercoaster of living with MG, I understand how important it is to be compassionate towards oneself. I have had moments of frustration, sadness, and even anger towards my condition. However, instead of suppressing these emotions, I have learned to acknowledge and embrace them. I have also learned to be kind and understanding towards myself, knowing that it's not easy to manage MG.

Shift from Guilt to Gratitude

One of the most powerful ways to practice self-compassion is to shift our mindset from guilt to gratitude. It's easy to feel guilty when living with MG—guilty for not being able to do as much as you used to, for having to ask for help, or for feeling like you are letting others down (which you are not!). However, this mindset of guilt only breeds negativity and can make coping with MG even harder.

Instead, we need to cultivate a mindset of gratitude. Be grateful for the abilities you do have, no matter how small. Appreciate the little victories, like getting out of bed on a tough day or mustering enough energy to do a favorite activity. Thank your body for what it can do rather than berating it for its limitations.

When I feel guilty about having to cancel plans or ask for assistance, I reframe my thinking through a lens of gratitude. Instead of focusing on what I can't do, I express gratitude for the people in my life who understand and support me through the challenges of

Dr. Liz Plowman

MG. Instead of feeling guilty for asking your spouse or care partner for help, be grateful that you have the support.

> **PRO TIP**: *Instead of, "I'm sorry to bother you," try, "Thank you for helping me."*

Cultivating a spirit of gratitude doesn't mean denying the difficulties of MG. It means choosing to focus on the positive aspects of your life, no matter how small they may seem. I'm thankful for the good days when my symptoms are more manageable. And I'm deeply grateful for the wisdom and resilience that living with this condition has given me. This mental shift can greatly boost your mood, outlook, and overall well-being.

Practice Self-Care

Self-care is a term that is often used in today's society, but what does it really mean? Essentially, self-care is an intentional and deliberate act of caring for your physical, emotional, and mental well-being. It's about prioritizing your needs and ensuring you are in a good place physically, mentally, and emotionally.

For someone living with MG, practicing self-care is crucial for managing the condition and maintaining a good quality of life. The first step towards self-care is to listen to your body and its needs. If you are feeling tired, take a break and rest. If you are feeling stressed, find ways to relax and unwind. If you are feeling overwhelmed, seek support from loved ones or professionals.

Another aspect of self-care is taking care of your physical health. This includes eating a balanced and nutritious diet, getting enough rest and sleep, and staying physically active within your limitations. It's also essential to follow your doctor's recommendations and take your medications as prescribed.

Self-care also involves taking care of your mental and emotional well-being. This can include practicing relaxation techniques such as deep breathing, meditation, or restorative yoga. It can also mean seeking therapy or support groups to help you cope with the emotional challenges of living with MG.

Set Boundaries

When living with a chronic condition like MG, it's essential to set boundaries and prioritize your needs. This means learning to say no to things that drain your energy or cause stress. It also means being assertive and communicating your needs to others.

Setting boundaries can be challenging, especially if you are used to prioritizing others' needs before your own. (Sound familiar?) However, it's crucial to understand that by saying no and setting boundaries, you are not being selfish. You are simply taking care of yourself and your well-being.

For example, if you have plans to attend an event but are feeling fatigued, it's okay to say no and prioritize rest. If you have a friend or family member who is not understanding of your condition, it's okay to set boundaries and communicate your needs to them. By setting boundaries, you are showing yourself the compassion and grace that you deserve.

Find Joy and Purpose in Life

Living with a chronic condition like MG can make you feel like your life revolves around managing your symptoms. However, it's essential to remember that you are more than your condition. You have passions, interests, and a purpose in life that go way beyond MG.

While managing your symptoms and conserving energy is crucial, it's also essential to make time for the things that bring you joy and fulfillment. This can be spending time with loved ones, pursuing hobbies or interests, creating beautiful artwork, or learning and professional development.

Finding joy and purpose in life has been a crucial aspect of managing my MG. I have become incredibly deliberate and intentional about choosing what I put on my proverbial plate and what I save my precious spoons for. I choose to prioritize my family, pursue my passion for writing, and serve the MG community by creating educational resources (such as this book). These activities bring me joy, fulfillment, and a sense of purpose outside of managing my condition. While writing this book has definitely cost me spoons, they were spoons that I happily spent to pursue something I am passionate about. And ultimately, that's what good energy conservation is all about—saving spoons to spend them deliberately and intentionally on things that really matter.

※

Living with MG is not easy, but it's essential to practice grace, compassion, and self-care to cope and thrive while managing this condition. By showing yourself grace, being compassionate towards yourself, practicing self-care, setting boundaries, and finding joy and purpose in life, you can live a fulfilling and meaningful life despite MG.

Remember to be patient and kind with yourself, and know that you are not alone in this journey. Surround yourself with a supportive network of loved ones, and seek professional help when needed. Most importantly, never forget that you are more than your MG. You are a strong, resilient, and amazing individual. Keep practicing good energy conservation skills, remember to take care of yourself, and spend your spoons on what truly matters.

You deserve it.

Acknowledgments

A few words of thanks...

First and foremost, thank you to my husband, Jason, for being my rock, my north star, and my calming presence. Your support is invaluable to me, and I couldn't do any of this without you. I love you.

I am immensely grateful to my business coaching team and accountability group. Your guidance, support, and the high standards you hold me to have been instrumental in my professional growth. You keep me on the mark, hold me to my deadlines, and inspire me to dream big. Thank you for believing in me and pushing me to be my best.

Thanks to my fabulous editor, graphic designer, and content reviewers. You made sense of my craziness and polished it beautifully!

And last but certainly not least, thank you to the *amazing* MG community for supporting me in my journey and allowing me to serve you. You inspire me every day!

Additional Resources

Thank you so much for taking the time to read this book. It means the world to me, and I hope it has been helpful to you on your journey!

❄

Before you go...

- For additional resources and a **downloadable content pack** to supplement this book, visit my website at www.lizplowman.com/spoons.
- For exclusive updates about my upcoming events, books, and classes, be sure to visit my website at www.lizplowman.com. You'll be the first to know about all the exciting things happening in my world!
- I'd love it if you'd follow me on social media! I post lots of educational and inspirational content that many people find helpful. Follow me on Facebook at www.facebook.com/themyasthenicpt and Instagram @themyasthenicpt.

About the Author

Dr. Liz Plowman, PT, DPT, OCS, TPS (Lt. Cmdr., Medical Service Corps, US Navy, Retired) is a physical therapist specializing in Myasthenia Gravis (MG) and chronic illness management. She is the owner of MG Physio and is dedicated to providing expert care and education for people living with MG. She has a keen interest in innovation and was an early adopter of telehealth physical therapy, even before it became popular during the COVID-19 pandemic.

She earned a doctorate in physical therapy (DPT) from Texas Woman's University and has a bachelor of arts (B.A.) and master of arts in teaching (MAT) from Austin College. She completed a residency in orthopedic physical therapy and a fellowship in pain neuroscience. She was an active-duty US Navy physical therapist until medically retiring in 2019 due to MG. At that point, she joined the faculty of the Texas Woman's University DPT program in Houston, Texas, and served as an Assistant Clinical Professor from 2019 to 2022. She has presented at numerous national and regional conferences and is a frequent guest speaker at local MG support group meetings and educational events. She has had multiple articles published in *Impact*, the magazine of the American Physical Therapy Association (APTA) Private Practice Section, and currently serves on the *Impact* editorial board.

Dr. Plowman's professional interests extend beyond the conventional realms of physical therapy. She is fascinated by pain science, rare neuromuscular disorders, psychologically informed care, and leveraging technology to enhance patient care and access. When not working, she enjoys traveling, learning new languages, cooking, writing, and SCUBA diving. She is an avid science fiction enthusiast, particularly anything related to *Star Trek*. She is still awaiting her admission letter to Starfleet Academy. And the Jedi Academy. And Hogwarts.

facebook.com/themyasthenicpt

instagram.com/themyasthenicpt

www.ingramcontent.com/pod-product-compliance
Lightning Source LLC
Chambersburg PA
CBHW032058020426
42335CB00011B/390